Coconut Cures

Preventing and Treating Common Health Problems with Coconut

Bruce Fife, N.D.

Foreword By
Conrado S. Dayrit, M.D.

Piccadilly Books, Ltd.
Colorado Springs, CO

Piccadilly Books, Ltd.
P.O. Box 25203
Colorado Springs, CO 80936, USA
info@piccadillybooks.com
www.piccadillybooks.com

Library of Congress Cataloging-in-Publication Data
Fife, Bruce, 1952-
Coconut cures /Bruce Fife.
p.cm.
Includes bibliographical references and index.
Contents: The Miracle Man -- The Fruit of Life - The Coconut Medicine Chest I:
Coconut Oil -- Coconut Oil on Trial -- Coconut Oil is Good for Your Heart --
The Coconut Medicine Chest II: Coconut Meat, Water, and Milk -- How to be
Happy, Healthy, and Beautiful -- Procedures, Formulas, and Recipes --
Remedies: An A to Z Reference.
ISBN 978-1-936709-15-1
1. Coconut oil--Health aspects. 2. Fatty acids in human nutrition. 3.
Coconut oil--Therapeutic use. 4. Coconut--Health aspects. I. Title.
QP752.F35F544 2004
615'.3245--dc22   2003070748

Printed in the USA

This book is dedicated to the memory of Paul Sores and his vision of spreading the knowledge of the healing properties of coconut throughout the world.

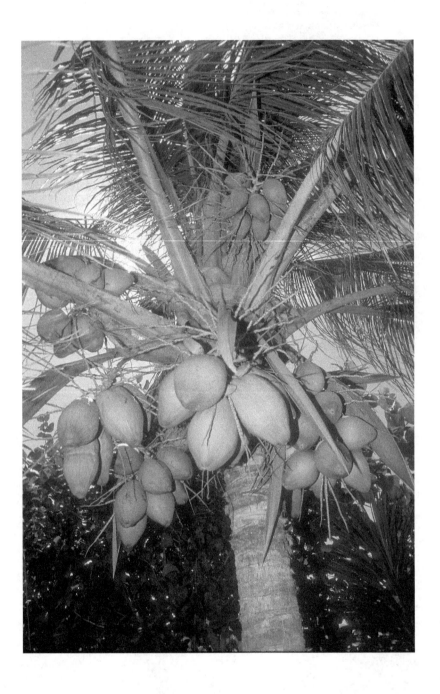

CONTENTS

FOREWORD

Conrado S. Dayrit, MD, FACC, FPCC, FPCP
Emeritus Professor of Pharmacology, UP College of Medicine

"If medium-chain triglycerides of coconut oil are good for prematures, infants and children, for convalescents, elderly and athletes, how can coconut oil be bad?" This intriguing observation of Dr. Bruce Fife set him on his search and eventual enlightenment on the real facts about coconut oil, hidden in journals that few physicians read. In this book, Dr. Fife's fourth on the virtues of coconut, he reviews the many varied health effects of coconut and in particularly coconut oil and the cures it can do.

The most remarkable property of coconut oil is that while it is a food, it also is an antibiotic, an immuno-enhancer, and a drug that regulates the body's function and defense mechanisms. It restores the normal balance of tissues of cells that have become "dysfunctional."

As a food, it is nutritious, safe and can be taken almost *ad libitum*. It provides energy and nutrition not only by itself but also by promoting the absorption of other foods particularly fat-soluble vitamins (A, D, E, and K) and minerals (calcium, magnesium, iron).

At the same time, it is a powerful drug that is non-toxic. It protects the body from infectious agents (viruses, bacteria, yeasts, fungi, protozoa, worms)—it can kill them. In other words, it is an antibiotic with the widest spectrum of action of all antipathogens. And it causes no harmful side effects. No resistance against it has been shown to develop. What a gift from Nature!

And this isn't all—it's just the beginning. Coconut oil is an immunoregulator, a defense regulator, and a function regulator. It makes the body work better, metabolize better, defend better, heal better. Chronic diseases like diabetes, asthma, atherosclerosis, hypertension, arthritis, Alzheimer's, autoimmune diseases like Crohn's, psoriasis, Sjogren's, even cancer, are subdued and become much easier to normalize, at lower doses or even suspension of usual therapies. All these disease conditions are inflammatory in nature.

Inflammation, characterized by various white cells attracted to a site of infection or derangement, is the body's mechanism for defense or for readjustment and healing. When successful, the inflammation subsides by itself. But when unsuccessful, as often is the case, the inflammation persists, becomes chronic, and eventually, becomes the disease itself producing the symptoms and complications.

How do we attempt to treat? We study the basic etiology, of course, and remedy that if we can. Most of the time, we fail and we treat symptomatically; we also try to reduce the inflammatory process (Vioxx tried that, caused inflammation elsewhere, and has now been withdrawn from the market). The body's inflammatory process is a very complex unbalancing (dysfunction) of pro- and anti-mechanisms, pro- and anti-substances (cytokines), whose various actions we are still trying to decipher. Interleukins (more than a dozen types), Tumor-necrosis factors (various types), interferons (also of various types), etc. are secreted by macrophages, polymorphonuclear granulocytes, T-cells, B-cells, killer cells, helper cells, plasma cells. The body has an arsenal that can make the U.S. defense forces green with envy. Unfortunately, we, owners of such a body, are still ignorant of what our Creator made for us.

So we go back to Nature for help. Here is the coconut tree and its fruit, the water, proteins and oil from its fruit, where Nature appears to have created another arsenal, a defensive arsenal for us, His creatures. Here are growth factors, anti-inflammatory factors, and regulatory factors ready for our use. There is now evidence for instance, that coconut oil inhibits (down-regulate is the modern term) pro-inflammatory cytokines (like IL-1, IL-6, IL-8) and stimulates (up-regulate) anti-inflammatory cytokines (like Il-10). This little finding gives us a little peek into why coconut oil can benefit such an unbelievably wide range of disease conditions.

"The drugstore in a bottle" is how coconut oil is now called in the Philippines where virgin coconut oil has been creating literally an "explosion" of the sick and not so sick treating every imaginable disease with this oil—and achieving, unbelievably rapid relief and cures. Success testimonials are coming by the hundreds, now thousands, emphasized significantly by "where can I get more of this virgin oil?" The supply can hardly catch up. Chapter 9 of this book is a wonderful A to Z reference of ailments curable by coconut oil and other coconut products.

Dr. Fife is asking for more testimonials. Here is one beauty not on his list yet: My cousin and classmate in UP Medical Class 1943 failed to attend our regular class reunions for some time because of his Sjogren's syndrome—a drying up of skin and mucous membranes—mouth, throat, nose, eyes, and rectal mucosa. He had to drink water for every swallow, he lacked saliva; he had to use eye drops every hour to lubricate his eyes, he had to lubricate his skin and lips with baby oil to prevent cracking. At one reunion, he managed to attend; I gave him some bottles of virgin coconut oil for him to take 3 tablespoonfuls daily. The other night he phoned me to say that he is now 80-90 percent improved. He eats well, regained his weight, his skin has regained its turgor, and his eyes need only 2 or 3 drops of lubrication a day. Coconut oil alone did this "miracle" in just two months.

This wonder oil was maligned for years as a contributor to heart disease because of its saturated fat content. The true fact is that the populations who take this oil daily in their food have little or no coronary heart disease—and no cancer, diabetes, or the other chronic ailments. The "My Battle with Cancer" story (Chapter 3) tells of a woman who developed a very malignant and resistant breast cancer. She had no family hereditary cancer history, avoided coconut oil and saturated fats and took only what her doctors advised her—hydrogenated soybean oil and corn oil. Are the "good" vegetable oils, chosen for the Food Pyramid Program the real culprits in America's on-going health crisis of diabetes, heart disease, Alzheimer's, and cancer?

Knowledge comes from successes and failures. How coconut oil kills germs and regulates body functions, or how it may fail to do so, needs intensive and extensive studies. There is a world of research to be done. In the end, we should understand a little better, not the mystery of life, but how we can live a healthier life, so that when we reach the end of our life span (120-140 years) we die healthy.

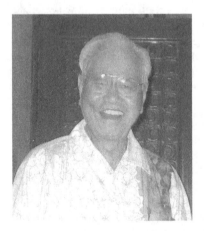

Dr. Conrado S. Dayrit is a cardiologist and an emeritus professor of pharmacology at the University of the Philippines. He is the former president of both the Federation of Asian Scientific Academies and Societies and the National Academy of Science & Technology. Dr. Dayrit has participated in many studies on the health effects of coconut oil and coconut oil derivatives. He was the first to publish clinical studies on the effects of coconut oil on HIV patients.

Chapter 1

THE MIRACLE MAN

As told to Bruce Fife by Jack DiSandro

Paul Sorse was one of the most remarkable men I have ever met. I'll always remember the time I was eating lunch in his little shop off Thames Street in Newport, Rhode Island. A man came crashing through the front door. "Where's Paul?" he cried grimacing in pain, his hands clenching a cloth dripping with blood. My appetite left as quickly as he entered.

The shop's owner, a slightly built, aging Filipino came out of the back room, "What's wrong?"

"I had an accident. My lawnmower cut my hand. You've got to do something!"

"Come over here."

Porfirio Pallan Sorse*, known as Paul to his friends, took the man behind the counter and examined the injury. The top of the man's thumb was hanging off to the side, attached only by a thin strip of skin. Luckily, the bone was not damaged. Paul lifted the top of the man's thumb and put it back in place, wrapped it in gauze, then soaked it in coconut oil.

"Keep the gauze moist with coconut oil and check back with me in a few days." Paul instructed.

A few weeks later I saw the man again, for he was one of Paul's regular customers. To my astonishment his thumb had completely healed. There wasn't even a scar.

Experiences like this were common. Paul had a long list of faithful customers who came to him for advice and treatment for a variety of health problems. Although he was not a licensed physician, people from all over came to him with their health problems. One middle-aged lady explained that she was plagued for years by a chronic skin condition, which the doctors were never

---

*Paul's last name, Sorse, is pronounced "sor-see."

able even to identify. The doctors gave her ointments, creams, and pills, but none of them worked. She was desperate and willing to try anything to bring relief. Paul instructed her to massage the affected areas of the skin with his oil. She began using it every day and to her amazement the problem disappeared just like magic. She became a devoted fan of his and continued to visit the shop to renew her supply of oil.

I, too, had a miraculous healing, of sorts, with his oil. On the back of my head was a hard growth, a cyst, the size of a quarter. My doctor wanted to surgically remove it, but before I let him do anything, I showed it to Paul. He told me to apply coconut oil to it with a little pressure. I was to keep applying oil to keep it constantly moist. I did this for several hours while watching TV. After a while it started to get soft and then all of a sudden, the liquid inside released through the pores and the lump was gone. No sign of an opening. It never came back.

At first I was amazed at some of the things I witnessed in Paul's shop and what customers told me. But in time, I became used to seeing miraculous cures. People from all over Newport would come to him to buy his coconut oil or to get treatment for some health problem. Paul's cures always involved the use of coconut oil. That's the only product he sold.

His fame as a healer, using only coconut oil, was known throughout the city. Several newspaper articles were written about him and his Copure (pure coconut) oil. A couple of large cosmetic companies approached him and offered to buy his secret formula for making the oil, but he refused to sell out. Running his own operation and controlling the quality of his product was more important than monetary gains.

He really believed in the healing power of coconut oil and wanted to help people more than he wanted their money. To him coconut oil was a panacea, useful for all illnesses and ailments. Many of his customers agreed.

I first met Paul about 25 years ago. He was in his late 70's at the time. I remember walking up to his little shop. On the outside was a sign that read: "Copure: Nature's Stone Aged Self Aid Remedy (Relieves all)." Another sign stated: "Copure—it feeds and lubricates nerve endings through the pores and relieves pain and aches instantly." Mangos and coconuts were lined up along the inside of the front windows. How strange I thought. Its unique charm invited me to enter.

The inside resembled a small deli. There were maybe three tables and a few chairs, a counter, and behind the counter a shelf holding a number of bottles filled with oil. In back were a small kitchen table, refrigerator, and a beautiful 45-year-old commercial cast iron stove with 10 burners and a large oven compartment. In the far back was a small room, about the size of a closet, containing a wooden cot. This is where Paul slept; his shop was his home. There was nothing elaborate or fancy about the place, he lived with only the bare essentials.

We became good friends. He would constantly talk, mostly about his coconut oil and how some day he would cure the world of illness. Paul never had any body odor or bad breath. What was amazing to me was that in the 25 or so years that I knew him, he never showered or took a bath with soap and water. Instead, every day he would massage himself with his oil from head to toe. He would drink a little of it and if he wasn't feeling good, he would drink a lot of it. His excellent health, physical condition, and virtually wrinkle-free face when he was in his 70's and 80's were indications of the effectiveness of his oil.

He didn't drink or smoke, but he ate almost anything, although he avoided most junk foods. He felt you could eat anything if your bowels were working properly and could move it out of your system quickly. He would say "clean the plumbing," and to do this he made a concoction of stewed prunes, coconut milk, apricots, and ginger. He would puree it and put it on desserts, ice cream, cake, or just eat it plain. It was delicious! He was a fabulous cook. Everything he cooked was incredible. I sure miss his cooking.

Although he was an excellent cook, and his shop somewhat resembled a little restaurant, he wasn't in the business of selling food. He often made a large pot of something to eat and kept it available for those who were hungry. Occasionally he would serve this to regular customers, close friends, or anybody who dropped by. Every day a blind man would find his way down Thames Street tapping his stick on the sidewalk until he came to Paul's place. Paul would prepare him a meal fit for a king. He did this every day for years and would charge the man a dollar or two. He had to charge something so the man wouldn't feel embarrassed. He did the same thing for an alcoholic who showed up now and then. Paul was small in stature, he only stood 5 feet 1 inch and weighed under 120 pounds, but he had a big heart.

Paul's business was coconut oil. That's where his real love was. All his conversations either started or ended with him talking about coconut oil. "The coconut is the king of foods, the mango is the queen," he would say. He would hold up a jar of oil, "The secret to good health is in this jar. There are millions of people all over the world dying of starvation and illness. It makes me sad to see this when I have the answer."

His place was clean and orderly. Whenever I entered, it either smelled of fresh coconut oil or some great meal he was cooking. It's no wonder many people ended up eating there.

Paul never advertised. He didn't have to. The oil sold itself. Once someone began using it, they were hooked. It was far superior to commercial creams and lotions and made an excellent cooking oil. As a healing ointment it was without comparison.

Paul relied totally on walk-in business, repeat customers, and word of mouth. His operation was small and his shop was rather empty compared to most stores bursting with goods and products. He had no employees.

Potential customers would wander into his place not knowing what they were walking into. When people entered, Paul would greet them with a friendly smile and start talking about his oil. He'd talk your ear off for as long as you were willing to listen about his sole cash product—Copure: all-purpose pure coconut oil. "It was good," he would claim, "for everything from cuts to colds, headaches, burns, sunburn, blisters, scratches, sinus, asthma, arthritis, rheumatism, aches and pains, stiff joints and muscles, pink eye, poison ivy, toothache, sore gums, and hardening of the arteries."

Paul would offer them a beverage of lemonade, ginger, and coconut milk. "Good for health," he'd say. "Not like Coke."

The oil sounded too good to be true and many people might have thought him to be just a snake oil salesman trying to put one over on them, but his friendly demeanor and hospitality soon won them over. He would have them try a little of the oil just to see how it felt. If the customer was hurting, he would give him a massage with the oil, at no charge. Often he would give potential customers a free sample and offer them some food along with his philosophy on life and health.

When he gave away a jar of coconut oil, he would tell them of its healing effects and encourage them to use their imaginations and to try it for any and all health problems. Over the years he built up a faithful following of customers. "I give much away," he says. "Knowledge multiplies as they tell others."

His stories were so intriguing, his food was so great, and his product so miraculous that people returned. He knew that once somebody began to use the oil they would discover for themselves how incredible it was and come back for more. That's why he was successful. The oil worked. If it didn't, his business could not have survived for the nearly 50 years in which he sold the product.

His customers came from all walks of life. Norma Taylor, a tennis pro, was a regular customer as was Dick Gregory, the humorist and political activist. Kathleen Cotta, who runs an herb farm in Portsmouth, would come in and buy two large jars of the oil; one for external use and one for internal use. "Believe it or not," she said, "I put it in tea or coffee. It's like vitamins."

Paul never marketed his product as a cure for any particular disease or health problem. His label read: "All-purpose pure coconut oil. For application to the skin and hair, external and internal daily use."

Those who used the oil would swear it was a panacea useful for most all illnesses and health problems. People would come and tell him how it relieved a certain condition or cured a particular health problem. Over the years he saw the oil work wonders. This is why he would rattle off a string of conditions the oil was useful for when potential customers wandered into his shop.

In the 1980s when President Ronald Reagan was having problems with hemorrhoids, Paul would say, "If he had my oil, he wouldn't have hemorrhoids."

As a body ointment, coconut oil is without compare. Paul would say it clears any skin disorder, even psoriasis. The skin must be kept constantly moist with the oil until the problem clears. He told me coconut oil would stop a wound from bleeding when applied with a little pressure. It prevents infection. When massaged over the entire body it helps regulate body temperature; if you have a fever it will lower your temperature. It relieves the itching, pain, and swelling of bee stings, insect bites, and poison ivy. It's excellent for burns and heals and prevents bedsores, eliminates wrinkles, acne and dandruff, and soothes chapped lips, sunburn, frostbite, diaper rash, and sore gums.

Used during or after pregnancy it can prevent stretch marks. A local gynecologist learned this fact from Paul and even now instructs all his patients with newborns to use coconut oil to eliminate stretch marks and revitalize the skin.

Paul said that the oil penetrates the skin through the pores, cleansing them and allowing the body to excrete waste. As the pores are discharging waste, they get clogged and create pimples, boils, etc. The oil penetrates the pores and melts the clogged waste. To demonstrate this he would have someone chew a stick of gum, then give him a teaspoon of oil. As he continued to chew with the oil, the gum would dissolve in his mouth. "This is what happens to the clogged pores," he would say. It upset Paul whenever he saw a girl with makeup on. He said makeup clogs the pores and causes wrinkles.

The oil seemed to work wonders on almost any skin problem. My wife had a large, dark mole the size of a pencil eraser on her chest. Paul told her she could get rid of it with his coconut oil. She was interested; nobody likes moles. He told her to apply coconut oil frequently to keep it moist. He said applying it once a day would eventually correct the problem, but it would work much faster if she kept the skin continually moist. She applied the oil every hour or two throughout the day just as he instructed. As the days went by, the mole started to shrink and began to develop pores or tiny holes. Eventually it just fell off. It was amazing!

I own two dogs. One of them developed a lump next to its eye. The veterinarian said it looked like a tumor and recommended immediate surgery because it was dangerously close to the eye. I figured if coconut oil was good for humans, it should be good for animals as well, so I began applying the oil to the lump on the dog's forehead. As time passed, the lump grew smaller and smaller and eventually disappeared. It never returned. We avoided the surgery.

Some time later my other dog developed sores on the bottom of his nose just above his upper lip. The vet gave him an antibiotic, but it didn't seem to do any good. After a week I stopped the medication and began to apply coconut oil to the sores. They got worse for a few days and then began to heal. He recovered without problem.

Paul wasn't surprised with the results, he told me coconut oil works for animals as well as people. His father used coconut oil on cattle after branding them. He did this to soothe the pain and help them heal faster.

The oil wasn't just for the skin. Paul would use it in all of his cooking. Every day he religiously swallowed a teaspoon of oil. It was like a tonic that kept him youthful both inside and out. It was also an effective medicine. "When taken internally," he would say, "it relieves stomach and intestinal ailments."

The oil was a tonic, a medicine, and a restorer of health. "It will make you happy, healthy, and beautiful," Paul would often say. He considered it a fountain of youth.

I would stop to see Paul just about every day for years. His coconut oil was as good as, or better than any on the market. I would pick up bags of coconuts from the wholesale produce place. They came 20 to a bag. Most of them came from Mexico. Sometimes the quality was good, sometimes poor, and naturally that would have an effect on the end result, but the oil would always do its thing.

It took Paul about three days to produce 4 to 5 gallons of oil, which was then fermented for another 30 days or so. I often helped him with the process. We would break the coconuts with a hammer, extract the meat from the shell with a screwdriver, grind the coconut in a meat grinder, cook it, cool it, press it, then simmer it in water all day, filtering it, waiting for the impurities to settle and the oil to rise, and finally, fermenting the oil for at least a month in sterilized jars. It was a tedious procedure, but every step was done with a reverence for the final product.

During the pressing phase of the operation Paul would use a hand-held potato masher. He would do this for hours on end to separate the oil from the water. One day I decided to help him squeeze the coconut. Paul was 82 at the time. I was comparatively young and healthy, but lasted maybe 15 minutes. My hands cramped, my forearms burned, and I had to quit. I told Paul there had to be an easier way. So one day when I went to pick up coconuts I saw a wine press; this was the answer. We bought a 50-gallon press and were able to get double the product with less wear and tear on Paul, to say the least. His son used the press for many years until he closed the business.

Paul's success as a healer and miracle man came from his exclusive use of one traditional medicine—coconut oil. Coconut oil has been used for thousands of years in the Philippines and the Pacific Islands. It is considered by these people to be "the cure for all illness." The coconut palm provides the staff of life for many Asian and Pacific Island populations. An ancient Filipino proverb says: "He who plants a coconut tree plants vessels and clothing, food and drink, a habitation for himself, and a heritage for his children." The coconut tree is the staff of life, yielding more diverse products for man's use than any other plant. For this reason, the coconut palm is highly valued in the Philippines and is called the "Tree of Life."

Porfirio (Paul) Sorse was born in the Philippines on October 2, 1895. He was the second child in a family of five. His father was a Baptist preacher. When parishioners got sick, his father would treat them with coconut oil, which was a traditional remedy used throughout the Philippines at the time. His father made the oil himself, using methods passed down from his father and his father before him. This is where Paul first learned to make fresh, virgin coconut oil.

During his early youth he worked on the family farm and in the rice fields. When the First World War came along, the U.S. Navy began to recruit Filipinos (the Philippines were a U.S. territory at the time). Young Sorse signed on as a cook. Paul served in the navy for three years. After the war ended he left the navy and joined the Merchant Marines working as a cook until 1925. Paul then moved to New York and lived in Greenwich Village with Filipino friends. His skills as a cook were sharpened while employed in such places as the Waldorf Astoria. He also worked for several wealthy families as a cook, driver, and handyman. He would cook wonderful meals, and take care of his employer's children, animals, and cars.

At one time he worked for the Chrysler family. On one occasion he said his boss told him he was pleased with his work and he would be rewarded for

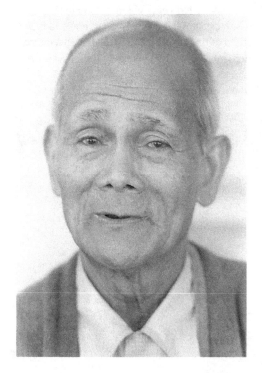

In 1995 Paul Sorse celebrated his 100th birthday. He was honored by the city of Rehoboth, Massachusetts as their oldest citizen. Still mentally sharp and physically active he made the potato salad and deviled eggs served to the guests who came to honor him.

it. A short time afterwards the man died in a private plane crash. He left to Paul what he described as a "large" sum of money. What a large sum of money was to Paul, I never found out. Knowing how frugal Paul lived, I doubt it was more than a few thousand dollars. To him this would be considered a substantial amount. Paul said he gave the money to a Filipino friend to go to Columbia University to become a doctor. He didn't expect his friend to pay him back. He told him that when he became a successful physician to use the money to help the Filipino people. That's the way Paul was, he always tried to help others.

Paul started making batches of coconut oil to help folks out when they were sick, just as his father used to do. His father's oil, however, was made using primitive methods and contained a high percentage of water, which caused it to go rancid within a couple of weeks. Paul improved on his father's original formula, eliminating all of the water, so that his had an indefinite shelf life, was smoother, and much easier to absorb through the skin.

When Paul retired in 1952, at the age of 57, he decided to market his coconut oil full time. "It's a helpful product, it meets human needs," he said. "It makes you happy, healthy, and beautiful. It goes through the pores, into the nerve centers. It helps you live a longer, healthier life." For the next 45 years he devoted his life to promoting the health benefits of coconut oil.

On March 28, 1998, Paul Sorse died at the remarkable age of 102. People that knew him said he looked and acted years younger than his age and remained physically active to the end, crushing and grinding coconuts to make his oil—evidence of the effectiveness of his product. Paul truly had discovered the fountain of youth. He is the most incredible man I've ever met. I miss him.

Chapter 2

THE FRUIT OF LIFE

FRUIT OF THE COCONUT PALM

The coconut palm is truly one of nature's natural wonders. It is reported to have 1,000 uses. Every part of the coconut palm is used for some purpose. From this tree you can derive everything necessary to sustain life. It is a source of food and drink to nourish the body, medicine to maintain and restore health, and materials to build shelter, clothing, and tools to provide the necessities of life. In India the coconut palm is referred to as "kalpa vriksha," which means "the tree which provides all the necessities of life." In the Philippines and the islands of the Pacific it is called the "tree of life."

Some people consider the coconut to be a nut while others call it a seed.* Those people who live in the tropics and use the coconut every day consider it a fruit—the fruit of the tree of life. Because of this and because of its nutritional and medicinal value the coconut can appropriately be called the "fruit of life."

In the tropics coconuts are a familiar sight. Coconut palms grow in abundance nearly everywhere. The coconut palm has come to symbolize the tranquility of an island paradise. Most people who live outside the tropics have never seen a living coconut palm. When they do, they expect to see the large, brown, hairy nuts they are accustomed to seeing in the grocery store. What they find is something quite different. Coconuts in their natural state are more than twice the size of those in the grocery store and are covered in a thick, smooth green or yellow husk. This husk is peeled and stripped off before shipping to markets overseas. The hard brown inner "nut" is what most people see in stores outside the tropics.

---

*Botanically the coconut is classified as a seed not a nut. It is the largest known seed in existence.

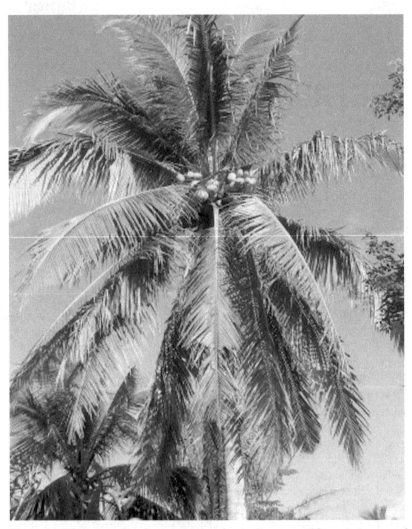

The scientific name for the coconut palm is Cocos nucifera. It is one of the most prolific and widespread trees in the world. It grows on islands and coastal areas in most all tropical climates. The coconut palm grows abundantly from the Tropic of Cancer north of the Equator (23 27' N) to the Tropic of Capricorn south of the Equator (23 27' S). In some places it grows beyond the tropics extending as far north as 26 degrees N in Central India and southern Florida to 27 degrees S in Chile and southern Brazil in South America. Although coconut palms do extend slightly outside the tropics they rarely bare mature fruit there. Coconut palms typically grow to 60 to 70 feet tall and have a life span of up to 70 years.

Unlike most fruit bearing plants, coconut palms produce year round and thus are always in season. Coconuts grow in bunches usually containing between 5 to 12 nuts, sometimes more. A mature coconut palm normally produces a bunch every month or 12 bunches a year. A productive coconut palm can yield 100 to 140 coconuts a year.

Coconuts take about 14 months to fully mature, producing a hard brown shell, some liquid, and a thick layer of white meat. The taste, texture, size, and content of the coconut meat and liquid varies as the nut matures. A very young coconut, less than 6 months old, is completely filled with liquid and has very little meat. At this stage the meat (endosperm) has a soft, jelly-like texture and can be eaten with a spoon. Both the liquid and meat are very sweet and delicious. Coconuts reach full size at about 6 to 7 months. At this stage they are only half developed and will take another 6 to 7 months to reach full maturity. As the coconut matures, the amount of liquid decreases and the meat increases in thickness and hardness. At about 10 to12 months the liquid to meat ratio is reversed. Fully ripe coconuts have only a small amount of liquid and a thick hard layer of meat. Both the meat and liquid become less sweet with age. Mature coconuts are the type most commonly found in grocery stores. In the tropics, however, young or green coconuts are among the most popular foods. Older coconuts are usually dried in the sun. Sun-dried coconut meat, called copra, is used to make oil. Fresh mature coconut meat is transformed into shredded coconut, coconut milk, or virgin coconut oil.

Young coconuts generally have light brown or tan colored shells as compared to the dark brown color of mature nuts. They are also much easier to crack open and eat. As coconuts mature the shells harden. Fully mature shells are very hard and difficult to break open. A hammer and a bit of elbow grease are often needed to crack open a mature coconut. With experience you can crack a coconut in half using the dull side of a machete with just a couple of blows.

Coconuts can produce a variety of edible products, the most common being meat, water, milk, cream, and oil. Other products include sugar, wine, and vinegar. Coconut meat is the white edible portion of the seed. It is generally sold shredded and dried. Fresh coconut meat can spoil quickly. When dried it can stay edible for many weeks and longer if sealed in an airtight container and kept cool, the way we usually see coconut sold in the store. Most shredded coconut has sugar added, but unsweetened coconut is also available, usually at health food stores. Coconut oil is extracted from fresh or dried coconut meat. The liquid inside a fresh coconut is often mistakenly called coconut milk but is actually coconut water. Coconut milk is completely different. There is a big difference between the two in taste, appearance, and nutritional content. Coconut milk is a manufactured product made by extracting the juice from coconut meat. Coconut water is clear or slightly opaque and looks almost like ordinary water. Coconut milk, on the other hand, is thick and white and looks just like cow's milk.

In addition to coconut meat, milk, water, and oil, the coconut palm yields many other edible products. The flower, which eventually transforms into the coconut, is the source of coconut sugar and coconut wine. The tip of an unopened flower is sliced off and the sap or toddy that flows is collected in bamboo or coconut shell containers. In the Philippines this sap is called "tuba." Up to a quart of sugary sap will drip out of the cut each day. Climbing to the top of the coconut palm to collect tuba takes a good deal of strength and skill. Apparently those who make the climb feel the rewards are worth the effort.

To make sugar, the sap is collected each morning and boiled in huge pots until it turns into a thick, sticky syrup which is then allowed to cool and harden. Because little processing is involved, the color, flavor, and sweetness varies from one batch to another. The color can range from a light tan to a dark brown. Depending on how long the sap was heated, it can be soft and sticky like taffy or hard like rock candy. It is often sold in crystallized chunks.

When we eat sugar and other carbohydrates they are converted into glucose and released into the bloodstream raising blood sugar or blood glucose levels. High blood glucose levels can have adverse effects on health. A scale called the glycemic index (GI) is used to gauge how quickly certain foods raise blood sugar levels.

Foods are assigned a number between 0 and 100 on the glycemic index scale. The number assigned to each food is determined by how quickly the carbs in that food raises blood glucose. The smaller the number, the less impact the food has on your blood sugar levels.

Glucose, taken orally, is very rapidly absorbed into the bloodstream and is assigned a glycemic index number of 100. All other foods are compared to pure glucose, with GI numbers between 0 and 100. A food that does not raise blood sugar at all has a GI of 0. Coconut oil has a GI of 0.

The presence of fat, protein, fiber, and acid (such as citric acid, lemon juice, and vinegar) in foods lower the glycemic index. Most foods are a combination of carbohydrate, fat, protein, fiber, and acid, so you cannot tell what the glycemic index is unless it has been tested. For example, when sugar (sucrose) is combined with other food ingredients such as a cream, nuts, and guar gum (a fiber used as a thickening agent), to make ice cream, the GI will be lower than the sugar alone.

Glycemic index testing carried out at the University of Sydney has determined that the glycemic index of coconut sugar is 54, which is relatively low in comparison to other forms of sugar.

The higher the GI, the greater the impact on blood sugar levels a food has. The GI is divided into 3 major levels:

There are many types of sweeteners and they each affect GI slightly differently. Coconut sugar is one of few sweeteners that fits into the "good" category of 55 or less. Below is the GI of some common sweeteners.

Sweetener	Glycemic Index	
Glucose	100	
Corn syrup	90	
Rice syrup	90	
Honey	87	
Molasses	68	
Sucrose	65	55 or less = low (good)
Maple sugar	54	56-69 = Medium
Coconut sugar	54	70 or higher = High (bad)

Fresh coconut sap is rich in vitamins and minerals and provides a valuable source of food in places where fruits and vegetables are limited, such as on volcanic atolls.

The sap ferments very quickly and within a couple of days in a warm tropical climate can contain 10 percent alcohol. This coconut wine is a traditional drink in many parts of the world. Sometimes it is distilled to increase alcohol content. In the Philippines this popular alcoholic beverage is called lambanog and resembles vodka or gin.

Because the water or juice inside the coconut is sweet, you might think it could also be fermented into alcohol. Coconut water has a lower sugar content than tuba and so produces very little alcohol. Fermented coconut water is usually used to make vinegar rather than alcohol.

COCONUT EVERY DAY

For generations people living in the coconut growing regions of the world have relied on coconuts for nourishment and health. These people quite literally use coconut in some form every day of their lives, and even benefit from it before they are born. Coconut is eaten to nourish the mother to assure a healthy baby and quick delivery. Expecting mothers massage the oil into their abdomen daily to ease childbirth and to prevent unsightly stretch marks. After delivery the oil is applied to tender areas to speed healing, and massaged on the breasts to soothe pain caused by nursing.

In Samoa the first food eaten by a mother after delivering her baby is a coconut dish called vaisalo. The vaisalo is made from young coconut meat and juice, with added starch to make it into porridge. The purpose of the vaisalo is not just to nourish the mother, but also to start her milk flowing quickly and abundantly. It is still widely eaten in Samoa, and not only by new mothers. It is eaten for breakfast and as a dessert.

From the first day of their lives babies are introduced to coconut oil. Mothers massage their babies thoroughly in coconut oil from head to toe. It is said to strengthen the muscles and the bones as well as prevent skin infections and blemishes. A few drops are always massaged into the soft spot on the baby's head. This is done in the belief that it helps prevent illness. When teething, babies' gums are massaged with coconut oil to relieve pain and speed healing.

In the islands the water from the inside of a fresh coconut is given to babies as a substitute for baby formula. Often infants are given both mother's milk and coconut water. If a mother can't nurse or if the infant has digestive problems, it is given coconut water from young coconuts. Infants have been raised from one or two months of age until weaning on little more than coconut water. The juice and meat from immature coconuts are used to wean babies off their mother's milk. The meat in young coconuts is soft and very tender, unlike the hard nut-like meat found in fully matured coconuts.

Coconut serves as a primary source of food for all ages in many island populations. The meat is eaten fresh, dried, roasted, and as a porridge mixed with coconut milk and water. In some areas coconut in one form or another provides most of the calories consumed each day.

In days past, and to some extent even today, children may wear very little clothing, but their bodies are always covered with coconut oil. Oil is applied after bathing, before going out into the sun, and before going out in the evening as protection from mosquitoes and sand flies. Everyone from the youngest to the oldest applies the oil over his or her entire body each day. It protects them from the rays of the hot tropical sun and keeps their skin young and healthy. It serves as an excellent moisturizer and suntan lotion. It is also applied to sores, rashes, cuts, and bruises. Coconut oil is always used to massage dry lips and for cold sores. It is warmed and poured into the ears, for earaches.

In Thailand, Sri Lanka, India and elsewhere, coconut oil is the primary oil used traditionally in cooking. Pacific Islanders, however, use coconut oil primarily for cosmetic and healing purposes. Most of the oil in their diet comes from coconut milk and cream. Almost everything is cooked in it.

The Samoans cook almost all of their food in a rich coconut cream. Even starchy fruits and vegetables are cooked in coconut cream. They eat coconut cream every single day and don't dilute the cream like many other Pacific Islanders do. On Sundays, in the earthen oven, Samoans cook their food; the only vegetable they usually eat are the leaves of the taro plant which they use to wrap undiluted coconut cream with onions and salt.

In the Philippines and elsewhere women put the oil in their hair after taking a bath. It has been observed that women who live in rural communities and still use coconut oil keep their beautiful dark hair even into old age, while those in urban areas where coconut oil is less frequently used tend to gray much sooner.

Coconut in one form or another is used as a source of nourishment, as a medicine, a protective and healing ointment, and a beauty aid. Quite literally the people use it from the day they are born until the day they die.

COCONUT IN TRADITIONAL MEDICINE

People from many diverse cultures, languages, religions, and races scattered around the globe have revered the coconut as an important source of both food and medicine. If you were in the Samoan Islands and became sick or injured, and were treated by traditional healers, part of your cure would involve the use of coconut. If you were in the coastal jungles of Central and South America and became ill, native healers would nourish you back to health using coconut. In the Philippines coconut oil is used to speed the healing of burns, cuts, and bruises. It is massaged into swollen joints and aching muscles and even used to speed the healing of broken bones. In East Africa you would be given a cup of palm kernel oil (similar to coconut oil) to drink. To them this oil is a health tonic and is the first medicine of choice among the native populations regardless of the illness.

In India, coconut in its many forms is used to treat a variety of health problems and nourish the body. Ayurvedic medicine has recognized the healing properties of coconut oil for over 4,000 years. The oil is valued for its antimicrobial properties, and the use of the oil in combination with herbs is widespread. Different preparations of coconut oil promote luxurious hair growth and protect the skin from infections and damage from sunburn. Dried coconut is used to expel parasites and improve digestive function.

Throughout the equatorial regions of the world where palm trees grow in abundance, coconut in one form or another is used to treat a diverse array of health problems with an amazing degree of success. Some of these conditions include: amenorrhea, asthma, bronchitis, bruises, burns, colds, colitis, constipation, cough, debility, dropsy, dysentery, dysmenorrhea, earache, erysipelas, fever, flu, gingivitis, gonorrhea, hematemesis, hemoptysis, jaundice, kidney stones, lice infestations, malnutrition, nausea, parasites, phthisis, rashes, scabies, scurvy, sore throat, stomachache, swelling, syphilis, toothache, tuberculosis, tumors, typhoid, ulcers, and wounds.

Before medically trained doctors were available, traditional healers took care of the people's medical needs. In the Philippines such a healer is called a *manghihilot*. Although modern medicine has taken over most of the medical care in the Philippines, manghihilots still tend to the needs of the sick and deliver babies in some rural areas of the country. Coconut oil serves as the basis for most of the cures used by the manghihilot. The oil is often combined with herbs such as garlic, ginger, and hot peppers and administered as needed. Manghihilots make their own oil from fresh coconuts.

Paul Sorse, whose story was told in the previous chapter, learned of the healing power of coconut from his father while growing up in the Philippines. He used that knowledge and expanded upon it. For over 50 years, he made and used coconut oil to heal the sick and injured and to keep himself and others as he would say, "happy, healthy, and beautiful." He called coconut the king of foods and considered it a cure-all and encouraged people to experiment by using coconut oil for any and all ailments. "It won't do any harm and may do a lot of good," he would say. He claimed that it is useful for treating burns, sunburn, blisters, cuts, scratches, eczema, insect bites, ringworm, piles (hemorrhoids), bruises, frostbite, pimples, colds, sinus infections, asthma, headache, arthritis, rheumatism, stiff joints, pinkeye, sore muscles, sore gums, toothaches, constipation, and wrinkles. He claimed it had unlimited uses. "There was no need to buy an individual product for each situation," he taught. Coconut oil could be used for many.

Paul's faithful following of customers testifies to the effectiveness of the oil. If it didn't work, they wouldn't have kept coming back. Paul believed all you need to do to be convinced of its usefulness is to try it. I agree with him. Just using it will demonstrate its effectiveness. Put it on your skin and see what a change it makes. It can make terribly dry, rough skin smooth and soft in a matter of a few weeks. Test it and see if your skin doesn't look and feel younger and healthier. I've witnessed it work miracles. What it does outside of the body, it can do on the inside as well.

Paul Sorse's life is a testimony of the effectiveness and safety of coconut oil. He drank the oil, used it in all of his cooking, and essentially bathed in it every day as he applied it from head to toe. It certainly didn't harm him, for he lived to be 102 years of age. It was probably the secret that kept him alive, healthy, and happy for so long.

THE COCONUT OIL SCARE

Although coconut has a long and respected history throughout the world, in recent times it has received an undeserved bad reputation. Coconut oil, in particular, has been labeled an artery-clogging saturated fat that should be avoided. Why? The answer to that question is a mixture of misconception, prejudice, and marketing. Because of the negative publicity that saturated fats have received in the past, many people are confused about the health aspects of coconut oil.

For over four decades saturated fats in general have been scrutinized because of their tendency to raise blood cholesterol. Coconut oil, being highly

Fibromyalgia

I have had very painful fibromyalgia for the past 15 years so I have been using the virgin coconut oil now for two months and have no pain at all, no pain!!!! And a lot more energy. And my skin has never looked so good.
Danne

Virgin coconut oil is the only thing that helped me with fibromyalgia. I was pretty sick when I started taking it and recommend it to every one that has body pain for any kind or to just build your immunity. I would say I started with positive benefits with 3 tablespoons day.
Eileen

Prostate

I have had a benign prostate enlargement for probably several decades. About 7-8 years ago it was so hard to urinate that I asked my doctor for some medicine. I took the medicine some years, and my nose was constantly blocked. Sometimes I tried without the medicine, and the nose opened! Then I read on the Net that a side effect of that medicine is breathing problems. So I changed to saw palmetto extract, which seemed to be as good as the medicine (Proscar).

I found out that the fatty acid composition of saw palmetto seed extract is somewhat similar to coconut oil, at least there are some common components. So I quit saw palmetto (which is expensive here in Finland) and have now for about 3 years relied solely on coconut oil. No problems urinating!
Iikka

---

saturated, has received the brunt of this criticism. In the mid-1980s the soybean industry sponsored a multimedia campaign to "educate" the public about the benefits of soybean oil and the dangers of saturated fat and coconut oil. Well meaning, but misguided, special interest groups such as The Center for Science in the Public Interest (CSPI) joined in on the attack on saturated fats. Together these groups succeeded in demonizing all saturated fats and particularly coconut oil. It was CSPI who coined the term "artery-clogging fat" in reference to coconut oil.

What the public didn't know at the time, and to be completely fair neither did CSPI, was that there are many different types of saturated fat, just as there are many different types of polyunsaturated fat. Each fat has a different effect on the body. Some saturated fats raise blood cholesterol, while others don't.

Coconut oil does not have a harmful effect on cholesterol. This fact was never mentioned in the anti-saturated fat campaign sponsored by the vegetable oil industry. People assumed that all sources of saturated fat were harmful. Before long everyone believed that coconut oil caused heart disease. Even health care professionals were confused. Several researchers who know the truth about coconut eventually stepped forward to set the record straight, but by this time the belief that coconut oil caused heart disease was so firmly established that people wouldn't listen. In fact, these researchers were actually ridiculed and criticized for defending coconut oil. So they backed off and remained silent. Food manufacturers sensitive to customer fear of saturated fats began removing coconut oil from their products. By the early 1990s coconut oil had virtually disappeared from the American diet and from the diets of many people around the world. Even in coconut growing regions of the world like the Philippines, coconut oil was avoided.

The truth about coconut oil remained hidden in medical journals, which few people read and even fewer understand. Many scientists who recognized the nutritional and medical potential in coconut oil continued with their research. While the public was being told about the dangers of coconut oil, the medical community was actively using it on their patients. Coconut oil, in one form or another, was and still is used in feeding tubes and IV solutions to treat critically ill patients. Coconut oil is a major ingredient in hospital and commercial baby formulas. It is used in over-the-counter medications and added to foods to protect them from spoilage. Nutritional products such as powdered sports drinks and energy bars use it. Few people, however, are aware of this. Often the terms MCT (i.e., medium-chain triglyceride, also known as fractionated coconut oil) or caprylic or lauric acids (the so-called artery-clogging saturated fats in coconut oil) were used to hide the fact that some form of coconut oil was in the product.

TRADITIONAL WISDOM

Coconut oil, meat, milk, and other products have been staples in the diets of the Asian, Pacific, and other island populations for generations. Over the past several decades people in the coconut growing regions of the world have been adopting Western foods and lifestyles; as a consequence, long held beliefs and practices have been fading away. As modern processed foods have become more available, traditional foods have become less popular. Like everyone else, these people have been influenced by misconceptions regarding coconut and particularly coconut oil. Believing it to be an "artery-clogging" saturated fat, coconut oil consumption and use has dramatically declined. In its place people eat margarine, shortening, and processed vegetable oils. Health problems such as heart disease and obesity that were unheard of a few decades ago when coconut was widely used are now common. This is especially true in urban areas where people are better educated and affected more by Western influences. Most of the newer generation have not been exposed to the traditional uses of coconut and know very little about it.

Fortunately, in many rural areas people still use coconut just as their parents and grandparents did. This is especially true among the poor, who can't afford the more expensive imported oils. These people have been able to enjoy the benefits of coconut and carry on the traditions of their ancestors.

As awareness of the nutritional and medical uses of coconut becomes better known, the use of coconut will find its way into more and more households. People from all walks of life and in all parts of the world will be able to benefit.

Activated Carbon from Coconut Shell

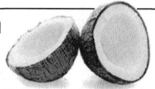

The hard shell of the coconut has many uses. It serves as a water container, serving cup, dish, spoon, ornament, and as fuel for cooking. One of the most beneficial uses it has is as a filter. When burned the coconut shell charcoal or carbon develops numerous tiny holes that allow it to absorb odors, toxins, and chemicals. Activated carbon coconut shell is a highly efficient medium for absorption and is used in gas masks, water filters, air filters, and even as a medicine.

Coconut shell becomes activated by creating numerous microscopic pores in the charcoal. One method of accomplishing this is to heat the coconut shell for several hours in a special kiln or furnace at 1650-2300 degrees F (900-1260 C) and pass steam through it. This process removes hydrocarbons and other volatile substances, creating a complex network of capillaries and fissures. The carbon is then crushed to produce a granular product.

Impurities and toxins are absorbed into these pores and trapped. Activated charcoal is used in a variety of products from cigarette filters to anti-pollution devices. It can also be purchased in a pharmacy or health food store as a detoxification or anti-poison over-the-counter medication. When swallowed the carbon absorbs toxins in the digestive tract.

Activated charcoal is more effective and easier to use than ipecac, a syrup that is often recommended for accidental poisoning that induces vomiting. Activated charcoal is the preferred method in hospitals for treating patients who swallow poison. It is also a convenient and effective home treatment if used within an hour after ingestion of a poison.

Chapter 3

COCONUT MEDICINE CHEST I: COCONUT OIL

The coconut, in a sense, can be viewed as nature's medicine chest. The products derived from it—meat, oil, milk, and water—can be used to nourish the body, prevent disease, heal injuries, and overcome sickness. When used with skill and judgment, these products have been useful in treating a wide variety of health problems. Many of the common health problems we encounter today can be prevented or alleviated by using the products from nature's medicine chest.

This subject is divided into two sections, The Coconut Medicine Chest I and The Coconut Medicine Chest II. In this and the following two chapters we focus on the health aspects of coconut oil. In the second section (Chapter 6) coconut meat, water, and milk will be covered.

The single most important thing that makes coconut one of nature's superior foods is the oil it contains. This is the reason why three chapters are devoted to it. Among the dietary oils, coconut oil stands out above all the rest in terms of its usefulness in food preparation and in medicine. In this chapter you will learn why coconut oil is different from other oils and why it is called the "healthiest oil on earth."

THE SECRET BEHIND THE OIL

Coconut oil is unique. It is unlike most other dietary oils. It is this difference that gives it most of its nutritional and medicinal properties. What makes coconut oil different from other oils is the fat molecules that make up the oil. All fats and oils are composed of fat molecules known as fatty acids. There are two methods of classifying fatty acids. The first, you are probably familiar with, is based on saturation. You have saturated fats, monounsaturated fats, and polyunsaturated fats. The second method of classification is based on molecular size or the length of the carbon chain within the fatty acid. You have short-chain fatty acids (SCFAs), medium-chain fatty acids (MCFAs), and long-chain fatty acids (LCFAs). When three fatty acids are joined together by a glycerol molecule you have a *triglyceride*. So you can also have short-chain triglycerides (SCTs), medium-chain triglycerides (MCTs), and long-chain triglycerides (LCTs). Sometimes people use the terms fatty acid and triglyceride interchangeably.

Short-chain fatty acids include butyric and caproic acids which have carbon chains containing four and six carbons respectively. Medium-chain fatty acids include caprylic, capric, and lauric acids with eight, ten, and 12 carbons. Long-chain fatty acids have carbon chains containing 14 or more carbons.

```
    H  H  H  H  H  H  H  H  H  H  H  O
    |  |  |  |  |  |  |  |  |  |  |  ‖
H–C–C–C–C–C–C–C–C–C–C–C–C–O–H
    |  |  |  |  |  |  |  |  |  |  |
    H  H  H  H  H  H  H  H  H  H  H
```

Lauric acid is a 12 carbon medium-chain fatty acid. It is the predominate MCFA in coconut oil.

```
    H  H  H  H  H  H  H  H  H  H  H  H  H  H  H  H  H  O
    |  |  |  |  |  |  |  |  |  |  |  |  |  |  |  |  |  ‖
H–C–C–C–C–C–C–C–C–C–C–C–C–C–C–C–C–C–C–O–H
    |  |  |  |  |  |  |  |  |  |  |  |  |  |  |  |  |
    H  H  H  H  H  H  H  H  H  H  H  H  H  H  H  H  H
```

Stearic acid is an 18 carbon long-chain fatty acid. It is one of the most common fatty acids in our food.

The vast majority of the fats in our diet, whether they are saturated or unsaturated or come from a plant or an animal, are composed of long-chain fatty acids (LCFAs). Soybean oil, corn oil, canola oil, olive oil, lard, and chicken fat, as well as most all other fats and oils in our diet, are composed entirely of LCFAs. Some 98 to 100 percent of the fat you eat each day consists of LCFAs, unless, however, you eat a lot of coconut or coconut oil. Coconut oil is unique; it is composed predominately of medium-chain fatty acids (MCFAs). It is the MCFAs in coconut oil that make it different from other oils and which give it its remarkable nutritional and medical properties.

Until recently coconut oil has not received much attention outside the research community. The reason for this is due to prejudice and a general misunderstanding about saturated fats. Many people, even now, are still confused about the different types of saturated fat. Many ill-informed writers continue to blindly lump coconut oil with lard and beef fat and label it an artery-clogging fat. But when you understand how coconut oil is metabolized by the body, it is easy to see that it does not contribute to hardening of the arteries or to heart disease. In fact, coconut oil can help *protect* you from heart disease. This topic is discussed more fully in Chapter 5.

Coconut oil is considered a "functional food," which means it possesses health benefits beyond its nutritional content. Medical researchers have been studying coconut oil for decades and have learned a great deal about this once maligned oil. The remainder of this chapter discusses some of the observed and documented effects of MCFAs found in coconut oil. References to medical studies are included to verify these statements and allow you to pursue further research on your own if you are interested.

DIGESTION AND NUTRIENT ABSORPTION

Medium-chain fatty acids, as the name implies, are shorter and smaller than long-chain fatty acids. The size or length of the fatty acid molecule is extremely important. Our bodies metabolize fatty acids differently depending on their size. Therefore, medium-chain fatty acids from coconut oil have a completely different effect on us than do the long-chain fatty acids that are more commonly found in our foods.

Because MCFAs are smaller than LCFAs, they digest much more easily and have a greater solubility in water. In fact, unlike LCFAs, pancreatic digestive enzymes and bile are not even necessary for their digestion. Because of this, coconut oil can provide a quick and easy source of nutrition without taxing the enzyme systems of the body.

Let me briefly explain how fats are digested and metabolized. When you eat foods containing long-chain triglycerides (LCTs), they are passed through your stomach and released into your intestinal tract. Almost all of the digestion of LCTs takes place in the intestine. Digestive enzymes from the pancreas and bile from the gallbladder are necessary for fat digestion. As LCTs are digested, the bonds holding the individual fatty acids together are broken. Individual fatty acids are then absorbed into the intestinal wall. Here they are packaged into little bundles of fat and protein called lipoproteins (chylomicrons). These lipoproteins are then funneled into the bloodstream where they circulate throughout the body. As they circulate, small particles of fat are released from the lipoproteins into the bloodstream. This is the source of the fat that collects in our fat cells and the source of the fat that collects in and clogs artery walls.

When medium-chain triglycerides (MCTs) are eaten, the process is different. MCTs also travel though the stomach into the intestinal tract, but

Fatty Acid Composition of Various Fats and Oils

	Fatty Acid	Coconut	Palm Kernel	Palm	Butter	Lard	Beef	Soybean	Corn
SCFA	Butyric (C4:0)*	-	-	-	3	-	-	-	-
	Caproic (C6:0)	0.5	-	-	1	-	-	-	-
MCFA	Caprylic (C8:0)	7.8	4	-	1	-	-	-	-
	Capric (C10:0)	6.7	4	-	3	-	-	-	-
	Lauric (C12:0)	47.5	45	0.2	4	-	-	-	-
LCFA	Myristic (C14:0)	18.1	18	1.1	12	3	3.0	-	-
	Palmitic (C16:0)	8.8	9	44.0	29	24	29.0	11	11.5
	Stearic (C18:0)	2.6	3	4.5	11	18	22.0	4	2.2
	Arachidic (C20:0)	0.1	-	-	5	1	-	-	-
	Palmitoleic (C16:1)	-	-	0.1	4	-	-	-	-
	Oleic (C18:1)	6.2	15	39.2	25	42	43.0	25	26.6
	Linoleic (C18:2)	1.6	2	10.1	2	9	1.4	51	58.7
	Linolenic (C18:3)	-	-	0.4	-	-	-	9	0.8
	% saturated	92.1	83	49.8	69	46	54.0	15	13.7
	% monounsaturated	6.2	15	39.3	29	42	43.0	25	26.6
	% polyunsaturated	1.6	2	10.5	2	9	1.4	60	59.5

*The C indicates carbon atoms. The number after the C and before the colon indicates the number of carbon atoms in the fatty acid chain and the number after the colon the number of double bonds. A 0 after the colon is a saturated fat, a 1 after the colon is a monounsaturated fat, and a 2 or 3 indicates a polyunsaturated fat.

Source: Applewhite, T.H. editor, Proceedings of the World Conference on Lauric Oils: Sources, Processing, and Applications. Champaign, Illinois: ACOS Press, 1994.

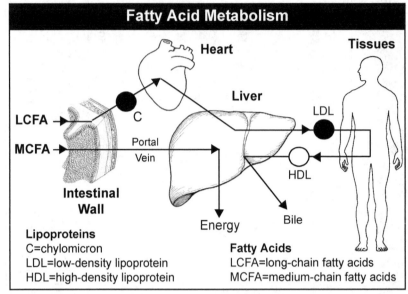

Fatty Acid Metabolism

Heart · Tissues · Liver · LDL · LCFA · MCFA · C · Portal Vein · HDL · Intestinal Wall · Energy · Bile

Lipoproteins
C=chylomicron
LDL=low-density lipoprotein
HDL=high-density lipoprotein

Fatty Acids
LCFA=long-chain fatty acids
MCFA=medium-chain fatty acids

Long-chain fatty acids are absorbed into the intestinal wall and combined with cholesterol and protein to form triglyceride-rich lipoproteins called chylomicrons. Chylomicrons are released into the bloodstream and are eventually transformed into low-density lipoproteins (LDL). LCFAs are circulated throughout the body as a component of lipoproteins. In contrast, medium-chain fatty acids are transported across the intestinal wall and into the portal vein where they are sent directly to the liver. In the liver MCFAs are used to produce energy.

because they digest so easily they are completely broken down into individual fatty acids by the time they leave the stomach. Therefore, they do not require pancreatic digestive enzymes or bile for digestion. As they enter the intestinal tract they are immediately absorbed into the portal vein and sent directly to the liver.[1] In the liver they are used as a source of fuel to produce energy. Therefore, MCFAs bypass the lipoprotein stage in the intestinal wall and in the liver. They do not circulate in the bloodstream to the degree that other fats do. Consequently, they do not get packed away inside fat cells or clog artery walls. They are used to produce energy, not body fat and not arterial plaque.[2-4]

Because MCTs are easily digested they also tend to improve the absorption of other nutrients as well. When coconut oil is added into the diet, it enhances the absorption of minerals such as magnesium and calcium, some of the B vitamins, the fat soluble vitamins (e.g., A, D, E, K and beta carotene), and some amino acids (i.e., protein).[5, 6] For instance, research demonstrates that symptoms of vitamin B deficiency are diminished when coconut oil is added to the diet. Signs of vitamin B deficiency in rats are counteracted when given coconut oil without any additional source of vitamins.[7] In young calves that are fed formula, adding as little as 2 percent coconut oil can prevent vitamin B deficiency.[8] Likewise, coconut oil improves calcium metabolism and bone health to the extent of preventing or counteracting the development of rickets.[9, 10] The oil itself does not contain all these nutrients, it simply makes what nutrients that are already in the diet more bioavailable.

Studies have shown that when low birth weight infants are given formula containing MCTs, they grow faster and have a higher survival rate. For example, in one study with two groups of low birth weight infants, coconut oil was added to the formula of one group. The group that received the coconut oil gained weight quicker than the group that did not. The weight gain was due to physical growth and not fat storage.[11] This must be one of the reasons why MCTs are naturally found in human breast milk.

MCFAs in human breast milk provide an easy source of nourishment as well as protection against infections. The more MCFAs in the milk, the healthier the baby is likely to be. The nutritional makeup and quality of mother's milk is determined by the types of foods the mother eats. If she eats poor quality foods, her milk will be lacking. If she eats a healthy diet her milk will provide the infant with all the nutrients it needs to be healthy and protect it from disease. If her diet includes a good source of MCFAs her milk will be enriched with these vital health-promoting fats. The MCFAs in human breast milk can be as low as 3 or 4 percent. When coconut products are included in the diet the levels of MCFAs can increase significantly. For instance, eating 40 grams (about 3 tablespoons) of coconut oil in one meal can temporarily increase the lauric acid in the milk for a nursing mother from 3.9 to 9.6 percent after 14 hours.[12] The content of caprylic and capric acids are also increased. Mothers who include coconut products in their daily diet can increase the MCFA content of their milk to as much as 18 percent. This increase would enhance the protective nature of the milk and provide a high percentage of easily digestible fatty acids that can promote growth and development. If the mother did not eat foods containing MCFAs before giving birth and does not eat them while nursing, her mammary glands will only be capable of producing about 3 percent lauric acid and 1 percent capric acid. Her child will lose a great deal of the nutritional benefits as well as the antimicrobial protection the infant could have otherwise had.

The following story illustrates the benefit of mothers taking coconut while nursing to enhance the nutritional value of their milk.

"I have a success story using virgin coconut oil! Last year I had my 9th baby. She didn't latch on well and we had some problems at the beginning with nursing, but since I'd nursed nearly all my children, I stuck it out and we worked out the problems. However, she wasn't really gaining weight like she should.

"All my other babies had been long and skinny, but growing on their own growth curve. My youngest, however, fell way off even the curve my others had typically followed. I was also dealing with postpartum depression. I finally went to our local naturopathic doctor when my baby was about 4 months old, and discussed the situation with him. He suggested several things for me to take, including virgin coconut oil. He told me that, in his opinion, it was very possible that since I'd had so many children, nursed most of them, and probably ate the typical American diet (which is unfortunately true), I could very easily not have enough *good* fats in my system and that could be affecting the quality of my milk.

"So, I bought a jar of virgin coconut oil and started taking it. Within 2 months, my baby had gained 3 pounds! Three months later at her next appointment, she had gained 2 more pounds. We're talking the difference between her gaining pounds versus ounces!

"My pediatrician was really surprised that she'd continued to gain in the same growth curve (even with learning to walk and everything), and asked me what I did differently to cause her dramatic weight gain. I wasn't sure how he'd react, but I told him about the virgin coconut oil and what the naturopathic doctor said. He sat there and nodded his head (no trace of attitude at all!) and wrote it in his chart. I was really impressed with how open he was.

"I'm even more impressed, however, with the virgin coconut oil. My baby's weight gain and her getting all the benefits of the virgin coconut oil through my milk is just flat out wonderful."

Nursing mothers and babies aren't the only ones coconut oil helps. Anyone with digestive problems can benefit by using coconut oil in place of other oils. Since digestive enzymes and bile are not necessary, those people who have enzyme insufficiency or gallbladder problems could benefit from using coconut oil. If a person has had surgery and had the gallbladder removed, digesting fats is a major concern. Fats are necessary for the proper digestion and absorption of many vitamins, minerals, and amino acids. If you have a digestive or gallbladder problem, adding coconut oil to your diet will greatly enhance the amount of nutrients your body will absorb.

Because coconut oil can provide a quick source of nutrition without taxing the enzyme systems of the body and because it enhances the absorption of nutrients in foods, it has been recommended in the treatment of malnutrition. A study conducted in the Philippines with malnourished preschool children showed coconut oil's superiority over soybean oil.[13] The children were divided into two groups. Each group was given identical meals except for the fat. One group was given soybean oil and the other coconut oil. At the end of 16 weeks the authors of the study reported that the group that received the coconut oil had "significantly faster weight gains and improvement in nutritional level." Because of its ability to make more nutrients available in the foods we eat, when you add coconut oil into your diet it is almost like eating a multivitamin and mineral supplement.

INCREASED ENERGY AND METABOLISM

Because MCFAs are preferentially used by the liver as a source of fuel to produce energy, coconut oil consumption can boost your energy level. It's like adding a premium grade gasoline into a high performance car. Your metabolism is shifted into a higher gear.

Adding coconut oil into your diet can help keep you alert and give you an energy boost to help with daily activities. Many people lack energy and quickly become fatigued. Coconut oil can help overcome this problem. Now the boost in energy you get from coconut isn't like the kick you get from caffeine, it's more subtle than that, but it's longer lasting. Unlike caffeine, the effects of coconut oil can last for many hours and you don't develop a dependence or addiction to it.

When I first was learning about the many benefits of coconut oil, I started using it myself. Although I had read in the medical literature about the studies on the influence MCFAs have on energy and metabolism, it really didn't hit me how much of an effect they really had. I remember taking some coconut oil in the evening a few hours before going to bed. When I went to bed at my normal time, I was full of energy, my eyes were wide open, and I couldn't go to sleep. I laid there for at least three hours before finally falling asleep. At first, I didn't know why I had so much energy. I didn't connect it to the coconut oil. A couple of days later it happened again. I took some oil in the evening and when I went to bed I had too much energy to sleep. It was then that I realized it must be from the coconut oil. Since then other people have reported similar experiences to me. I now refrain from eating coconut oil late in the evening.

What a great natural alternative to coffee! Instead of drinking coffee to wake you up in the morning or keep you going through an exhausting day, a little coconut oil can do the same thing, but without the side effects of caffeine. A tablespoon of coconut oil in a cup of warm herbal tea, cocoa, or juice can boost your energy.

The effects of MCFAs in coconut oil have been so impressive that researchers have investigated their use for enhancing endurance and athletic performance.[14, 15] Results of many of these studies have been encouraging but mild when compared to drugs. In Australia horse trainers are feeding their racehorses coconut cake containing about 10 percent coconut oil. They claim this enhances the horse's performance. Because it doesn't have a drug-like effect, coconut oil can legally be used in athletic competition. For this reason, coconut or MCT oil is frequently added to powdered sports drinks and energy bars. Even if you're not an athlete you can enjoy the energy boost you get from coconut oil. Who wouldn't like to have higher level of energy throughout the day to help them accomplish more without feeling tired or exhausted? People who lack energy or suffer from chronic fatigue can greatly improve their lives by adding coconut oil into their diets.

Energy

I took the oil for the first time yesterday, 2 tablespoons. I did not notice anything until this morning. I am 60 years old. And the last year I have had trouble waking up and I feel fuzzy. This morning before I even opened my eyes (5 am) I knew something was different. My head was clear and balanced and I could have jumped right out of bed but I lie there a while just enjoying it.
Ruth

I have been using coconut oil for our whole family and no other oils for the past several months! I no longer have cravings for sugar and I have lots of energy.
Susan

I have been consuming coconut oil for about 6 weeks and have lost about 5 pounds. I have noticed an increase in energy. I had low metabolism since I was a teen. I am now 76 years old. I walk for an hour three times a week and the day before yesterday I felt so good that I walked for two hours and felt good.
Sally

I started taking coconut oil faithfully six weeks ago. I am up to 2 ounces a day and I am experiencing fabulous results… I feel great and have much more energy. I am a massage therapist and have a very busy practice. I have been tired and burned out for years, but still I plugged away and satisfied my customers. I have not felt tired for weeks now.
Bruce

I started using coconut oil three weeks ago and immediately my energy level (which was quite low from my hypothyroidism) increased by approximately 600 percent. Wow! I feel 10 years younger.
Noah

WEIGHT MANAGEMENT

Because MCFAs are used to produce energy rather than packed away into fat cells, coconut oil can be useful in weight management. In fact, coconut oil has gained the reputation as being the world's only natural low-calorie fat. A low-calorie fat is a strange concept, but coconut oil fits that description. It has this reputation primarily for three reasons. First, coconut oil actually has fewer calories than any other fat. All other fats have 9 calories per gram. Coconut oil has slightly less, about 8.6 calories per gram. That isn't much of a difference, but this isn't the main reason for coconut oil's low-fat reputation. The other two reasons are much more important.

The second reason is that coconut oil satisfies hunger better than any other fat, and probably any other food. When you add coconut oil to a meal, you become satisfied sooner and do not get as hungry between meals so you can go longer without snacking. By the end of the day you tend to eat less food and consume fewer calories. This means you have fewer excess calories that can be packed away into storage as body fat.

A study published in the *International Journal of Obesity* illustrates this effect.[16] The study compared the effect on hunger between MCTs and LCTs. It consisted of three phases of 14 days each. Volunteers had access to high-fat foods for each of the 14-day periods. In the first phase the diet contained 20 percent of fat from MCTs and 40 percent LCTs. In the second phase there were equal amounts of each. In the third phase there was 40 percent of fat from MCTs and 20 percent from LCTs. The subjects were allowed to eat all they wanted in each phase. Researchers found that as MCTs content in the food increased, total food consumption, and consequently calorie consumption, decreased. Coconut oil, which is composed predominately of MCTs, can satisfy hunger faster and longer than any other dietary oil.

The third reason for coconut oil's reputation as a low-calorie fat is that it lifts metabolism to a higher level. As metabolism increases, calories are consumed at a higher rate. Since more calories are burned up, fewer are left to be converted into body fat.

Metabolism is evaluated by measuring energy expenditure. Energy expenditure is the rate at which calories are consumed. The higher the metabolism, the higher the rate of energy consumption. Just adding coconut oil to a meal will essentially reduce the effective number of calories in the meal. In a study that measured energy expenditure before and after a meal containing MCTs, energy expenditure in normal weight individuals increased by 48 percent. In other words, metabolism increased by 48 percent. In obese individuals energy expenditure increased by an incredible 65 percent![17] So the more overweight a person is the greater an effect coconut oil has on stimulating metabolism. This is good news for overweight individuals who want to use coconut oil to help them lose weight.

More good news is that this increase in metabolism doesn't last for just an hour or two after a meal. Studies have shown that after a single meal containing MCTs, metabolism remains elevated for a full 24 hours![18] So after eating a meal containing coconut oil your metabolism will be elevated for 24 hours. During this time your body will be burning calories at an accelerated rate and you will enjoy an increased level of energy.

Weight Loss

One of the best things is that I am no longer getting the "I'll kill if I don't eat something NOW" hypoglycemic hunger hurricanes. I got on the scales this morning and was delighted to discover I had dropped 6 pounds! This is exciting.
Alice

When I started I weighed 316 and wore a size 52 pants. When I got on the scale this morning I weighed 256 for a total loss thus far of 60 pounds and I'm in 44's now...People that I work with intermittently comment on how much energy I have now. My 20-year-old son is doing this with me and has gone from 203 to 177 in three months. I don't count calories and in fact I think at any intake less than 2500-3000 I'd loose weight. I do figure out the calories every couple of weeks just to make sure I don't slip below 2000 a day. And I have a tendency to do that because I am never hungry anymore. With the fat intake at this level I am usually satiated for nine hours or so and find it very easy to inadvertently skip a meal if I get busy.
Chuck

Over the last 20 years I have been steadily and gradually gaining weight. You couldn't call me fat—but there I was, just too wobbly in all the wrong places. This year I decided to do something about it—finally. I went on a fruit diet. Nothing happened. I tried the cabbage soup diet (without the meat). Nothing happened. I fasted for a week. NOTHING HAPPENED!

That was when this book (*Eat Fat, Look Thin* by Bruce Fife) came into my hands—a godsend. I stopped fasting and began eating food again, but using coconut oil. After a few days I weighted myself—I had lost 5 pounds! Since then I have lost a total of 24 pounds, and still losing steadily at about a pound a week, enjoying full meals.
Sharon

Researchers at McGill University in Canada have determined that if you replaced all the fats and oils in your diet that are made of LCTs, such as soybean, canola, safflower, and other typical cooking oils, with an oil composed of MCTs, such as coconut oil, you can lose up to 36 excess pounds a year![19] You can experience this amount of weight loss without changing your diet or reducing the total number of calories you consume. All you need to do is simply change your oil. Because of these effects, coconut oil is not only being recommended as a means to manage weight but also as a means to treat obesity.

I have had many people come to me and report how they have lost 5, 10, 20 pounds or more by simply adding coconut oil to their diets. One lady wrote to me and said she had been using coconut oil for a year and a half and in that time she had lost 56 pounds! On the other hand, some people complain that they have not been successful in losing weight. The results you experience will vary depending on other factors such as diet and activity level. If you sit around eating candy and donuts and gorge yourself at mealtime, coconut oil isn't going to do the impossible. To achieve the best results in weight management coconut oil should be used in conjunction with a sensible diet and exercise program. Add the oil to meals to help satisfy hunger and prevent overeating and enjoy the energy boost it gives. For people who want a safe and natural way to lose weight I recommend my book *The Coconut Ketogenic Diet* (previously titled *Eat Fat, Look Thin)*. In it I discuss how to use coconut oil for weight loss, how to stop food cravings, and how to feel satisfied so you don't get hungry between meals.

Because of coconut oil's effect on weight loss, some people have asked the question: "Will it make skinny people skinnier?" From what I've seen, the answer is no. Studies have shown that the less body fat you have, the less effect coconut oil has on stimulating metabolism and burning up calories. Also, people who are underweight and malnourished gain weight and become healthier when coconut oil is added into their diets. So it appears that if you are overweight, coconut oil helps you lose excess fat, but if you are underweight it helps you gain. Whether you are overweight or underweight, coconut oil added to the diet will help you reach the size that is healthiest for you.

THYROID FUNCTION

Low thyroid function is becoming one of our most prevalent health problems. Doctors who specialize in thyroid health estimate that up to 40 percent of the population is affected to some degree. Thyroid problems can affect the health and function of every cell and organ in the body. The reason for this is because the thyroid gland regulates metabolism. When thyroid function decreases, all processes in the body slow down. Digestion slows down, healing and repair slows, immune system response slows, hormone and enzyme production slows, body temperature drops, etc. Everything functions at a lower rate of efficiency. Consequently, chronic health problems begin to arise. Symptoms associated with low thyroid function include the following:

Overweight	Itchiness
Cold hands and feet	Food intolerances/sensitivities
Fatigue	Brittle nails
Migraines	Slow healing from injuries
PMS	Bruise easily
Irritability	Heat and cold intolerance
Fluid retention/swelling	Hypoglycemia
Anxiety and panic attacks	Frequent or persistent colds
Severe depression	Frequent urinary tract infections
Decreased memory	Frequent yeast infections
Lack of concentration	Depressed immunity
Low sex drive	Joint pain
Low body temperature	Poor coordination
Constipation	Irregular menstrual periods
Insomnia	

If you have three or more of the symptoms listed above, you may have a low thyroid problem. A combination of factors can contribute to the development of hypothyroidism including genetics, diet, lifestyle factors, and illness (e.g., autoimmune disease, cancer, etc.). If low thyroid function is not related to genetics or illness, it might respond to lifestyle and dietary changes. If so, coconut oil may exert a significant influence in correcting the problem.

Our body's metabolism has basically three settings—fast, medium, and slow. Metabolism shifts between all three during the day depending on different circumstances. At times our body functions best at high speed, while at other times it prefers to go slow. Most of the time it runs in neutral or medium, not too fast and not too slow.

Metabolism will shift into high gear in response to certain circumstances. For instance, when we are involved in physically demanding activities our need for energy increases so metabolism gears up. Also, if we get an infection and become sick, metabolism increases to accelerate production of antibodies and speed healing and repair.

Metabolism shifts into low gear when we sleep or rest or when food consumption decreases. When we fast or even diet, the body interprets it as a period of starvation. In response, metabolism slows down to conserve energy to ensure survival during the time when food is less plentiful.

A normal, healthy body constantly shifts in and out of all three levels of metabolism. When conditions that cause the body to gear up or gear down are over, metabolism rebounds back to normal. This is the way it's suppose to work.

However, because of certain circumstances, the body can become stuck in low gear. It can stay stuck for weeks, months, or even years. Subsequent events that shift the metabolism into low gear can crank metabolism down even lower. If metabolism doesn't recover before a new episode hits, it can sink lower and lower. As metabolism slows down, body temperature decreases. This is why some people may have a temperature only slightly below normal while others may be off by two or three degrees.

What causes metabolism to get stuck in low gear? A combination of both stress and malnutrition can be the cause. When we are under stress the body responds by increasing its metabolism. If you have to take an important test, run a race, or meet a deadline at work, the body responds by pumping up metabolism. As metabolism increases, cellular processes are shifted into high gear. The demand for energy to fuel these activities is increased. The need for vitamins and minerals is increased because the enzymes that run all chemical activities in the body depend on these nutrients. So vitamins and minerals are used up at an accelerated rate. If there are plenty of nutrients in storage, and if the stress is removed after a brief period of time, the body is perfectly able to cope with this shift in metabolism.

A problem arises, however, when stress becomes chronic or severe and the body is undernourished, as are most people who eat a lot of overly processed or junk foods. Frequent or very severe stress places a great demand on the body for vitamins and minerals. If the needed nutrients are not present, the body senses a situation similar to that of starvation and shifts into low gear. When nutrients become depleted the body goes into a state of exhaustion and becomes locked in low gear. It does this as a means of self-preservation to conserve energy and nutrients that are vital to maintaining life.

If enough nutrients are not supplied to adequately replenish the body's storehouse, metabolism remains stuck in low gear. Repeated episodes of stress drive metabolism even lower, making it harder to recover. What types of stress can bring about this situation? Any type of chronic or severe physical, mental, or emotional stress, such as pregnancy and childbirth, divorce, death of a loved one, job demands, family troubles, surgery, accidents, illness, or lack of sleep.

Malnutrition, or rather subclinical malnutrition, is very common in our society. Eating sweets, refined grains, and processed vegetable oils that have been stripped of much of their natural vitamins and minerals have created a society of people who are on the edge nutritionally. Pregnant women have an increased demand for good nutrition. The unborn child demands ample nutrients for proper growth and development and will steal them from the mother's body if they are not supplied in her diet. If she doesn't eat properly, her own nutrient reserves can become dangerously depleted. Add the fact that pregnancy can be a very stressful time, nine months of stress culminating in several hours of arduous labor and childbirth. It is no wonder why 80 percent of those with low thyroid function are women.

The first step in correcting a thyroid problem caused by excessive stress and poor nutrition is to improve nutritional status. Cut out junk foods, eat more fresh fruits and vegetables, take a multiple vitamin and mineral supplement, and start using coconut oil daily.

Since MCFAs boost metabolism, coconut oil has a stimulatory effect on the thyroid. In a sense, it can kick start the thyroid gland so that it runs at a higher level of efficiency. If the body receives proper nutrition, thyroid function can return to normal.

Many people have reported how simply adding coconut oil into their diets has stimulated metabolism as evidenced by an increase in body temperature. Normal body temperature is 98.6 degrees F (37 degrees C). It is normal for

---

Low Thyroid

It's only been about three months since I've begun using coconut oil. My skin is like a newborn babe's. My face is lovely and rosy. The bottoms of my feet are like a teenager's (I don't rub it in, I merely ingest it). For the first time in 53 plus years I am WARM as long as I use the coconut oil. And I've lost 11 pounds. My hair is beautiful! As far as I'm concerned virgin coconut oil is my miracle food.
Linda

I bought some oil for the health benefits, and started it today, as soon as I got it. My temperature (taken as experiment to see if the oil did raise it) the last few days has been 97.2 to 97.6 and after taking the oil it rose to 98.8 and 98.3 later on in the day. Have to admit this really surprised me, despite having read of it, and I'm really looking forward to seeing if it stays up and how else it affects me.
Carole

I have the autoimmune version of hypothyroidism and I now have lots more energy after using it for several weeks, which cannot be said for anything else I have tried. To me it is a blessing.
Suzanne

Since I started taking the coconut oil my temperature has come up and pretty much stayed in the 98.7 range! And, it's only been 2 weeks...I have more energy and feel like myself again!
Rachel

Arthritis, Insomnia, and Irritability

During the past several months, I have been experiencing severe insomnia. I do not believe in taking drugs to assist in sleeping, but it had gotten so bad that I got a prescription from my doctor. On using the prescription (and I have only tried this a couple of times) I was still only able to increase my nights sleep from about two hours to about four and after taking the sleeping pills I felt so much worse the next day that I had abandoned that as a solution to my problem. I have noticed that since using the coconut I am now getting a full eight hours sleep.

Also, the pain in my hands, vertebrae, and knees from arthritis have almost completely disappeared. I still have the occasional twinges in the knuckle in the little finger on my right hand, but I suspect that is because it has calcified.

I almost feel foolish writing this, because I cannot quite believe that I have been the beneficiary of such incredible improvement from all my ails, just from consuming coconut milk and oil. I keep expecting the problems to return. Another benefit is that I have lost the chronic irritability that I have had for so long that I was beginning to think that I have had a personality change. I can only attribute all of these things to the coconut oil as nothing else about my life has changed.

Rhea

I must say I noticed a GREAT change in arthritis symptoms. I had some swelling and discomfort in one of my knees for approximately 3 months prior to starting the daily consumption of virgin coconut oil. When I heard about the virgin coconut oil, I purchased some and rubbed it around the knee area where the swelling was; my knee immediately stopped hurting and the swelling has gone away. I've not even had an inkling of the symptoms of pain in my knee since taking the virgin coconut oil.

Chris

temperature to vary by about 1 degree throughout the day, being lowest in the early morning and late evening. Temperatures below this indicate low thyroid function. People with chronic mid-day temperatures of below 97.6 degrees F (36.4 degrees C) have reported it rising to normal levels with daily coconut oil consumption. When used regularly in combination with a nutritious diet, some have been able to reduce or completely get off thyroid medications. I have worked with people who have been hypothyroid for over 20 years, required thyroid medication, had chronically low temperatures, and suffered with most of the symptoms listed on page 40. After coconut oil therapy they experienced dramatic improvement in their symptoms, no longer needed medication, and now have normal body temperatures. For more information on how to use coconut oil to stimulate metabolism, boost energy, and improve thyroid function, I recommend my book *The Coconut Ketogenic Diet*.

CELLULAR FOOD

Coconut oil provides a source of highly efficient cellular food. MCTs do not require pancreatic digestive enzymes or insulin for their digestion, utilization, and conversion into energy. Relatively little stress is placed on the enzyme and hormonal systems of the body. Cells are able to get nourishment quickly and efficiently even when conditions such as diabetes or pancreatic insufficiency exist.

Your state of health is a reflection of the health of your cells. If your cells are sick, you will be sick. If only a fraction of the cells in you liver were sick and malfunctioning, your liver would be sick and less efficient. Likewise, your overall health will suffer. However, if all the cells in your body were healthy, you would be healthy too.

Eating foods containing coconut oil is one way of giving your cells a source of quick, easy nourishment, thus helping them to remain alive and active. MCFAs can give cells a needed energy boost, increasing metabolism to help them expel waste and toxins, utilize life-giving oxygen, and perform at top efficiency. As the cells inside your body become healthier, you become healthier.

All your cells, whether they are on the inside or the outside of your body, are able to absorb MCFAs to produce the energy they need to power biological functions. The miracles they work inside the body also occur on the outside. This is one of the reasons why coconut oil can work wonders for skin problems. Coconut oil is one of nature's most remarkable healing salves. All it takes to convince someone of the effectiveness on the skin is to try it. It makes skin look and feel younger and healthier. Blemishes such as acne, eczema, psoriasis, fungal infections, wounds, and sores dramatically improve in many cases. Even precancerous skin lesions and moles begin to fade with regular use.

You can think of coconut oil as food for your skin. When it is applied topically, the cells absorb the MCFAs and convert them into energy. Metabolic activity increases, stimulating healing and repair. Skin problems and blemishes disappear. This may be why coconut oil is so useful for cuts, burns, ulcers, and other skin and tissue injuries.

I am constantly amazed at the reports I hear from people who begin using coconut either internally or externally. Numerous chronic health problems seem to fade away with regular use. One of the most incredible effects I frequently hear is how coconut oil reduces swelling and chronic pain. Laura and Bonnie's stories below are typical.

"Because of a motorcycle accident when I was 22 (now 51) my leg and knee has always been a problem," says Laura. "Especially with age the problem has worsened. Since I work on the computer for hours on end, the knee and leg tend to swell and cause lots of pain. Upon getting up and trying to walk after being seated for so long, it is hard to even walk…that is until the virgin coconut oil. For some reason, after taking it for about 5 or 6 days, I noticed when getting up to walk the knee was not swollen as before and best of all, *no debilitating pain!*"

"I use to be a runner/jogger," says Bonnie, "but the last year or so my knee began swelling and I couldn't bend it enough to run anymore. About a month after starting the virgin coconut oil the swelling went down to almost nothing."

Inflammation, aches, and pains of all types including arthritis, back pain, and fibromyalgia all seem to lessen or vanish when people begin to use coconut oil regularly. The reason isn't fully understood yet, but part of it I'm sure is because the oil is used as food to feed and energize the cells. There is evidence that suggests that coconut oil has a mild anti-inflammatory effect.[20] Inflammation is almost always associated with chronic pain and sometimes is the cause. Another reason for the oil's healing effect is that it appears to increase circulation (see the section on diabetes in Chapter 5). Consequently, the healing process is enhanced and pain and swelling are relieved.

ANTIMICROBIAL

If you asked me what natural means you could use to prevent or even cure an infectious illness, my answer would be to try coconut oil. Coconut oil? Yes. Coconut oil is one of the best natural remedies you can use for infectious illness. With nothing more than coconut oil I've seen chronic skin fungus healed in a matter of days, bladder infections vanish in less than two days, and people recover from the flu within as little as 12 hours.

One of the most remarkable characteristics of medium-chain fatty acids in coconut oil is their ability to kill germs and parasites. When we eat MCTs they are transformed inside our bodies into monoglycerides and medium-chain fatty acids, both of which possess powerful antimicrobial properties capable of destroying disease-causing bacteria, fungi, viruses, and parasites.

Years ago researchers discovered that human breast milk contains MCTs. These medium-chain triglycerides play a vital role in the health of developing infants. Not only do they provide a source of nutrition, but also protect the baby from a wide variety of infectious illnesses. In fact, research has shown that the presence of MCTs in mother's milk is the primary ingredient that protects newborn infants from infections for the first few months of their lives, while their immune systems are still developing.[21]

The MCTs in coconut oil are identical to those in human breast milk and possess the same antimicrobial properties. For this reason and others, coconut oil or MCTs are routinely added to hospital and commercial baby formulas. Medical research over the past 40 years has shown that MCFAs from coconut oil kill bacteria that cause such things as stomach ulcers, urinary tract infections, pneumonia, gonorrhea, and other illnesses.[22-27] They kill yeasts and fungi that cause ringworm, athlete's foot, and candidiasis.[28] They destroy viruses that cause influenza, herpes, measles, mononucleosis, hepatitis C, and even kills HIV—the AIDS virus.[29-35] Coconut meat and oil can kill or expel parasites such as tapeworms, lice, and giardia.[36-38]

Tracy Jones, a natural health practitioner in Hawaii, uses coconut with much success in his practice. "One recent case in particular is kind of interesting," he says. A mother of a 4-month-old infant girl with the symptoms of pinworms visited his office. "The infant had eruptions covering its entire head—very nasty looking." She told him that her doctor was unable to do anything for her baby. The infant was too young to try to feed it coconut oil directly. However, the mother was breastfeeding. He reasoned that if the mother consumed the oil her milk would be enriched in MCFAs, which might help with the infant's condition. He gave the mother some coconut oil and told her to eat three tablespoons a day along with some coconut water. The mother returned a couple of days later. The eruptions that had once covered the infant's entire head were dramatically reduced. The woman said on the previous day her daughter vomited some nasty looking white stuff and then vomited again only this time it had a lot of black specks mixed in it. Parasites? Possibly. The baby was doing much better and was now sleeping through the night for the first time. He told the mother to massage coconut oil into the remaining eruptions on the baby's head and to continue eating the oil. When she returned a few days later the infant had only a small red spot the size of a quarter remaining on her head and appeared to be in good health. "Not bad, eh?" he says. "Her mother will be using the coconut oil from here on."

The antimicrobial properties of MCFAs were first reported by Jon Kabara, Ph.D. in 1966. His initial studies were aimed at solving food preservation problems. MCFAs, which are foods in themselves, provided a harmless means to keep food products free from invading fungi, bacteria, and viruses.

When medium-chain triglycerides in human breast milk or coconut oil are consumed, our bodies break them down into monoglycerides and free fatty acids. As explained earlier in this chapter, triglycerides are simply three fatty acids linked together by a glycerol molecule. As triglycerides are broken down in the digestive tract, the fatty acids are removed one by one. When one fatty acid is removed, the remaining glycerol and two fatty acids become a diglyceride. If two fatty acids are removed leaving only one fatty acid attached to the glycerol, this is a monoglyceride. If all three fatty acids are removed, only the glycerol is left. The fatty acids, since they are now detached, become free fatty acids.

Triglycerides and diglycerides do not show any antimicrobial effects, monoglycerides and free fatty acids do. Coconut oil is composed entirely of triglycerides. So coconut oil does not exhibit antimicrobial activity. Its antimicrobial properties become activated only after the triglycerides are converted into monoglycerides and free fatty acids in the digestive tract.

The three important medium-chain fatty acids in coconut oil are lauric acid (C12), capric acid (C10), and caprylic acid (C8). The monoglycerides of these fatty acids are monolaurin, monocaprylin, and monocaprin. All of the medium-chain fatty acids and their monoglycerides exhibit antimicrobial activity. Monolaurin, the monoglyceride of lauric acid, has the greatest *overall* antibacterial, antiviral, and antifungal effect. Each, however, has a different effect on various organisms. For example, one may be more effective at killing *E. coli* than another but less effective than the other against *Candida albicans*. All of them work together synergistically to provide the widest and strongest germ-killing effect.

The microorganisms that appear to be most vulnerable to MCFAs and their monoglycerides are those encased in a lipid (fat) membrane—lipid coated viruses and bacteria. These organisms depend on host lipids for their own structural components. MCFAs and monoglycerides are absorbed into the organism's outer membrane. These fats have a destabilizing effect which weakens the membrane to the point that it disintegrates and falls apart, killing the organism. This process is so effective it can kill even the supergerms that have become resistant to antibiotics. Bacteria cannot develop resistance to this type of action, so MCFAs can be used repeatedly without fear of the organisms developing antibiotic resistance and evolving into so-called supergerms.

Most of the research has been done in vitro or in laboratory settings. However, more recent in vivo or clinical research on animal and human subjects is verifying these studies. In animal studies coconut oil has shown to reduce protozoa (single-celled parasites) in the digestive tract.[39] Coconut preparations have been used successfully in India to treat tapeworm infestations.[40] Clinical studies currently in progress using pure coconut oil as well as monoglycerides derived from coconut oil are showing good results in treating many infectious conditions.

Research indicates that coconut oil may be a promising natural remedy for a large number of infectious diseases, even serious ones such as AIDS and SARS. As far back as the 1980s researchers discovered that MCFAs in coconut oil could kill HIV—the AIDS virus. As reports of coconut oil spread, many HIV infected individuals began adding it to their treatment protocol. This led to many anecdotal accounts of HIV patients experiencing partial or complete recovery.

The first clinical test of coconut oil on HIV patients was carried out at the San Lazaro Hospital in the Philippines in 1999.[41] Fourteen HIV patients between the ages of 22 and 38 completed the study. None of them could afford or ever received anti-HIV treatment. The study lasted for 6 months. Treatment benefit was defined as reduction in viral load (a measure of the number of viruses in the blood) and increase in CD4 count (a measurement of the number of white blood cells). Subjects received the equivalent of 3½ tablespoons or less of coconut oil daily. Some of the patients received pure coconut oil while others received monolaurin, which is the monoglyceride of lauric acid in coconut oil.

By the end of the study eight of the 14 patients had a decreased viral count, which is good. Five had an increased CD4 count, which is also good. Eleven subjects regained weight, again a good sign indicating improvement in health. According to Conrado Dayrit, MD who participated in the study, "This initial trial confirmed the anecdotal reports that coconut oil does have an antiviral effect and can beneficially reduce the viral load of HIV patients."

The AIDS organization, Keep Hope Alive, has documented several cases in which HIV/AIDS patients have reported marked improvement in health after consuming coconut oil, coconut meat, or coconut milk. In some cases all evidence of the infection was removed. For example, one man dropped his viral load from 600,000 to non-detectable levels in 2½ months by eating a bowl of coconut and cooked cereal every day along with a healthy diet containing lots of fresh fruits and vegetables.

In a second case a person with a viral load of 900,000 ate half a coconut a day. After 4 weeks, his viral load dropped to around 350,000. After the second month, his viral load remained the same and his doctor added the drug Crixivan to his protocol. After 4 weeks, his viral load dropped to non-detectable levels. Unlike the first case cited above, this person ate a typical American diet that included ample amounts of junk food. His progress probably would have been quicker if he had a better diet.

Case number 3. A man consumed ¾ can (10 ounces) of coconut milk daily for 4 weeks. His viral load for HIV dropped from 30,000 to 7,000. He used no other antivirals. He also used some of the other immune based therapies like Naltrexone and Thymic Factors. He reported a doubling of his T cell counts (both CD4 and CD8) during the 4-week period.

Case number 4. A person with CFIDS who was 36 pounds underweight reported his CD8 and CD4 counts doubled and that he gained 15 pounds after

---

Infections

I have had a huge improvement in my sinus and chronic ear infections. I put some in my nose every day and in my ears. I only take one tablespoon a day at this point. I normally have three to four sinus infections a year and 5-7 ear infections a year. For the past 6 months of taking virgin coconut oil I have had NONE, even with swimming!
Lori

I have Hepatitis C and after taking virgin coconut oil for 6 months and then had my viral load checked it was so low it was almost undetectable. Coincidence? I doubt it.
Nancy

Because of the nature of my job, I come into contact with a large number of sick people. This is especially true during the cold and flu season. Since I started using coconut oil regularly about two years ago I noticed a drastic decline in the frequency and intensity of the common cold and the flu in myself. If I do happen to find myself infected with the flu virus I take one tablespoon of coconut oil every 3 hours until symptoms are gone. I have done this several times. The longest it took was 32 hours and the shortest was 12 hours.
Joe

INFECTIOUS DISEASE

Published medical studies show that MCFAs in coconut oil kill bacteria, viruses, fungi, and parasites that cause the following illnesses.

Bacterial Infections
Throat and sinus infections
Urinary tract infections
Pneumonia
Ear infections
Rheumatic fever
Dental cavities and gum disease
Food poisoning
Toxic shock syndrome
Meningitis
Gonorrhea
Pelvic inflammatory disease
Genital infections
Lymphogranuloma venereum
Conjunctivitis
Parrot fever
Gastric ulcers
Septicemia
Endocarditis
Enterocolitis
Acne

Viral Infections
Influenza
Measles
Herpes
Mononucleosis
Chronic fatigue syndrome
Hepatitis C
AIDS
SARS

Fungal Infections
Ringworm
Athelete's foot
Jock itch
Candidiasis
Diaper rash
Thrush
Toenail fungus

Parasite Infections
Giardiasis

3 months. He eats 2 whole raw coconuts weekly along with taking dietary supplements. He avoids fried foods, eats lots of vegetables, and reports he is doing much better.

Case number 5. A man on an immune based therapy reduced his viral load from 60,000 to 800 within 6 weeks after consuming one can (14 ounces) of coconut milk daily. Fourteen ounces of coconut milk contains about 5 tablespoons of coconut oil.

Case number 6. A man was taking an anti-HIV drug cocktail that included Crixivan, AZT, and 3TC along with dietary supplements. Using this therapy his viral load was reduced and kept steady at 2400, but he continued to lose weight and his health deteriorated. He added 3 tablespoons of coconut oil daily to his diet. Some weeks later he quit taking the drugs. After three weeks on the coconut oil his laboratory test showed his viral load was unchanged, but he was feeling better. Usually when individuals stop taking anti-HIV drugs their viral load quickly returns to previous high levels. Coconut oil apparently helped to keep his viral load under control.

MICROORGANISMS KILLED BY MEDIUM-CHAIN FATTY ACIDS

Medical research has identified a number of pathogenic organisms that are inactivated by medium-chain fatty acids in coconut oil. Below is a listing of some of the organisms reported in the medical literature.

Viruses
Human immunodeficiency virus (HIV)
SARS coronavirus
Measles virus
Rubella virus
Herpes simplex virus (HSV-1 and -2)
Herpes viridae
Sarcoma virus
Syncytial virus
Human lymphotropic virus (Type 1)
Vesicular stomatitis virus (VSV)
Visna virus
Cytomegalovirus (CMV)
Epstein-Barr virus
Influenza virus
Leukemia virus
Pneumonovirus
Hepatitis C virus
Coxsackie B4 virus
Parainfluenza virus type 2

Bacteria
Listeria monocytogenes
Helicobacter pylori
Haemophilus influenzae
Staphylococcus aureus
Staphylococcus epidermidis
Streptococcus agalactiae
Escherichia coli
Pseudomonas aeruginosa
Acinetobacter baumannii
Neisseria
Chlamydia trachomatis
Streptococci Groups A, B, F, & G
Propionibacterium acnes
Gram-positive organisms

Parasites
Giardia
Ciliate protozoa

Although MCFAs are powerful enough to kill potentially deadly organisms such as HIV, they are harmless to us. In fact, our cells use them as food. So they feed our cells but kill deadly invaders. How incredible! This shows the wisdom of nature and how a simple food can both nourish and protect. This is one of the reasons why coconut oil is regarded as a functional food—a food with health benefits beyond its nutritional content.

Even relatively large amounts of MCFAs in the diet are harmless to us. It just provides our cells with more food to fuel metabolism, growth, and repair as well as kill invading germs. Jon Kabara, Ph.D., professor emeritus of chemistry and pharmacology at Michigan State University, has been studying the effects of MCFAs on human health for 50 years. He states, "It is rare in the history of medicine to find substances that have such useful properties and still be without toxicity or even harmful side effects." Medium-chain triglycerides are so safe that even a newborn baby can eat them without harm. After all, they are an essential component of mother's milk.

Parasites

I passed a worm yesterday. It can only be attributed to taking the coconut oil in earnest for the last three weeks. It was quite thrilling to see because that sucker was alive!

I also want to emphasize that my health is excellent as I've been into the health movement since the '70s. Also my hygiene is impeccable. So if I have worms, guess what, so does nearly everyone else.

Marilyn

My husband was very sick. He couldn't say it hurts here, or I have a cold or the flu or a fever. It was just a general feeling of not being well and it never went away. I thought that he might have cancer. He did not have the energy to get out of bed, and had a low tolerance for "children noise" and life was hard. So I really delved into books to find help. A sample sent to an "alternative medicine" place told us he had hookworms all over his digestive tract full of viruses and bacteria. We first tackled the parasites, and we did Essiac tea and lots of nutritive stuff, and herbs as well as the liver flushes and kidneys cleanses. Well he got well and I regained the husband I married. However, over the months that followed we noticed that the parasites must have come back. My husband's stomach began to hurt again about 6 months later, my gingivitis came back, children who had stopped wetting the bed started again, etc. We do have dogs, cats, horses, cows, goats, geese, chickens, etc. And I have two little boys who play outside in the frog pond and the dirt and suck their thumbs. So we wormed again and 6 months later again. But this past summer my husband decided to just make sure he got his recommended dosage of coconut oil and see if that would take care of things. He is one of those people who is steadfast and diligent. So he has never missed a day and slowly over the course of time the pain in his stomach has gone away and his energy has again returned. This is great news to me, because it means that rather than "worming" my family a couple of times a year, if I keep the coconut oil in their diet we may stay clean.

Annette

Although MCFAs can kill a large number of disease causing organisms, they don't kill *all* microorganisms. They may not be effective for some infectious illnesses so you can't expect coconut oil to be a cure all. This is actually a good thing. Unlike antibiotics, which kill all the bacteria in the body, MCFAs do not. They leave the good bacteria in the gut unharmed. One of the drawbacks with antibiotic treatment is that friendly gut bacteria are killed too. These bacteria are necessary for good health. They produce important nutrients such as B vitamins and compete with harmful organisms, such as candida—a single celled fungus. If the good bacteria are killed by antibiotic use, candida can overrun the intestinal tract causing candidiasis. This is an often overlooked health problem that generally goes unrecognized but leads to many health problems and is very difficult to correct. Some people battle with chronic systemic candida infections for years.

Unlike antibiotics that are only good against bacteria, MCFAs are effective in killing bacteria as well as viruses, fungi, and parasites. MCFAs and more specifically their medium-chain monoglycerides not only kill many disease-causing microorganisms but evidence suggests that they enhance the immune system.[42] Therefore, they can be of benefit against most any infectious disease. Since coconut oil is a food, you can eat it every day to help keep illness away.

DIGESTIVE DISORDERS
Intestinal Environment

Inside each of us live a vast number of bacteria—about 100 trillion in all. They outnumber all the cells in the body and are comprised of over 400 species. Most of them live in the digestive tract. About one third of our fecal matter is bacteria.

For the most part, these bacteria are not parasites; they are lifelong companions to which we owe our lives. Without them we could not survive. Within days after birth our digestive tract is teeming with microscopic life. These "friendly" microbes create an environment inside our bodies that provides us nourishment, protects us from illness, and facilitates proper intestinal function. They manufacture vitamins such as niacin (B-3), pyridoxine (B-6), vitamin K, folic acid, and biotin. They manufacture the enzyme lactase, which is necessary for digesting milk and dairy products. They produce antibacterial substances that kill or deactivate disease-causing bacteria, viruses, and yeasts. Some bacteria have anticarcinogenic properties that protect us from cancer.

Coexisting along with the good bacteria, however, are organisms that can cause us harm. As long as we provide the friendly bacteria a reasonably good diet and avoid using certain drugs, they greatly outnumber the unfriendly microbes and keep them from causing trouble. If for some reason the bad organisms are allowed to grow out of control, they can cause a variety of symptoms ranging from annoying to fatal. Conditions associated with an imbalanced environment in the digestive tract include frequent infections, constipation, diarrhea, candidiasis, psoriasis, eczema, acne, allergies, headaches, gout, arthritis, cystitis, colitis, Crohn's disease, irritable bowel syndrome, chronic fatigue, irritability, depression, hormonal imbalances, ulcers, and some forms of cancer. It may be surprising to learn that an overgrowth of unfriendly organisms in the digestive tract can cause so many problems and affect so many different parts of the body.

One of the most troublesome organisms in our digestive tract is the yeast *Candida albicans*. Candida provides a good example of how the overgrowth of an unfriendly organism can affect the health of the entire body. Yeast is a single-celled form of fungus. Candida lives in the digestive tract and normally doesn't cause any harm because its numbers are kept relatively low by the immune system and friendly bacteria. However, if allowed to proliferate, it can become a real troublemaker. Many women are all too familiar with vaginal yeast infections. Parents may have encountered it in the form of thrush, a candida infection in the mouth and throat of infants, or as diaper rash, a candida infection of the skin growing under the moist environment of a diaper. When candida infects the entire body it causes candidiasis.

Normally candida and other disease-causing microbes are confined to the digestive tract. While these organisms may not produce symptoms themselves, their waste products—mycotoxins and exotoxins—can be very toxic. *Myco* means fungus, *exo* means bacterial, and *toxin*, of course, means poison. These poisons pollute the body and put the immune system under a great deal of stress. Energy is continually being sapped as the body works feverishly to counter the effects of these toxins. A lack of energy and chronic fatigue are often the result. Seasonal illnesses become frequent and recovery is prolonged. How many bouts with colds or flu have you had this year? If your digestive system is in perfect condition you shouldn't have any.

An overgrowth of disease-causing microbes can physically damage the lining of the intestinal wall, creating a whole new set of health problems. Just as an infection can cause a festering sore on the skin, the same type of problem can occur in the digestive tract. These localized infections may be evidenced as ulcers.

Candida is especially insidious because it is capable of changing its form if allowed to grow. If left unchallenged, candida converts from a single-celled form into a multi-celled or mycellial fungal form with hairy, root-like projections called rhizoids. These rhizoids penetrate into the intestinal wall. When candida or bacteria penetrate the intestinal wall it affects the intestines' ability to absorb vitamins, minerals, amino acids, and fatty acids, leading to nutritional deficiencies. As the intestinal wall becomes perforated it allows bacteria, toxins, and undigested food to pass across the intestinal barrier and enter the bloodstream. This condition has been called leaky gut syndrome. Even relatively harmless bacteria, if allowed to enter the bloodstream, can cause infections. This often results in chronic low-grade infections and inflammation that can lead to a number of symptoms and feelings of ill health. Undigested proteins from our food are allowed to pass through the intestinal wall and migrate into the bloodstream. The immune system identifies these food proteins as foreign invaders and initiates a frantic attack, resulting in allergy symptoms. So your food allergies may be caused by an imbalance in the microbial environment of your digestive tract. The entire body is affected by the health of the digestive tract. The health of the digestive system is so important to our overall health that many natural health practitioners believe that *all* chronic health problems originate in the intestines.

What causes an imbalance in the environment of the intestinal tract? Diet is a primary culprit. As long as you feed the good bacteria and keep them alive and thriving, the bad organisms don't have a chance to work their mischief. What do good bacteria like to eat? They prefer foods rich in fiber—vegetables, whole grains, legumes, and coconut—the same types of foods that are good for our bodies. Candida and other harmful microbes prefer simple carbohydrates—sweets and refined flour products. Cakes, cookies, candy, white bread, sugary drinks, and the like feed candida and promote their growth. These are the foods that harmful organisms thrive on and the foods that are the least healthy for us. Not surprisingly, the diet best suited for people is also best for friendly bacteria.

Certain drugs, especially antibiotics, promote the growth of troublesome microbes. Antibiotics kill friendly bacteria just as efficiently as they kill disease-causing bacteria. Steroids (cortisone, ACTH, prednisone, and birth control pills) also cause damage to friendly bacteria. Yeasts are not harmed by antibiotics or steroids. When the good bacteria die off, candida is allowed to multiply unrestrained. This leads to yeast overgrowth. Symptoms may or may not be manifested immediately. If they are, it is generally as a vaginal yeast infection but may also be expressed as a skin rash (skin fungus). A single course of antibiotics or steroids can upset the balance in the intestinal tract that can last indefinitely.

The best way to fight off candida and other destructive microbes is to help reestablish the good bacteria. You do this by eliminating foods that feed candida and eat a high-fiber diet. Coconut meat is very high in fiber and helps feed the good bacteria. The MCFAs in coconut oil kill candida and other disease-causing organisms, but do not harm friendly bacteria. A source of probiotics such as yogurt, kefir, or cultured coconut can help reestablish the beneficial bacteria. MCFAs are also used as food by the cells in the intestinal wall. The fatty acids are absorbed into the cells and used as fuel to power metabolism. When used topically on the skin, coconut oil is very effective in promoting the healing of damaged tissues. Conceivably, they can help to heal the perforations in the intestinal wall caused by bacteria and yeast that make the gut leaky. Eating coconut and coconut oil daily can be a great aid in reestablishing and maintaining a healthy intestinal environment.

Ulcers

An ulcer is an open sore on the skin or a mucous membrane. It may be shallow or deep and is usually inflamed and painful. Ulcers can occur anywhere along the digestive tract. Canker sores and cold sores are ulcers that occur in or near the mouth; peptic ulcers occur in the stomach or duodenum (upper portion of the small intestine); ulcerative colitis occurs in the small or large intestine (colon).

Ulcers may be the result of a number of factors. Although the exact cause for many ulcers is still not clear, stress and infections appear to be major contributing factors. Stress lowers our resistance to infections, making us more vulnerable to organisms that can cause ulcers. Cold sores, for example, are caused by the herpes virus; canker sores are often associated with hemolytic streptococcus bacteria. Cancer can also initiate open sores. Skin ulcers can develop in basal cell carcinomas, which are a form of skin cancer. Likewise, some ulcers that occur in the digestive tract are caused by cancer.

At one time, excessive stress was believed to be the primary cause of peptic ulcers. Stress stimulates the secretion of gastric acid in the stomach. Without food to act as a buffer, it was believed that the acid burned holes through the lining of the stomach causing the ulcers. It is now known that peptic ulcers are caused by a bacterium called *Helicobacter pylori*. While stress is no longer considered the primary cause, it may still be involved by lowering resistance to infection.

A bland diet and antacids are often recommended for peptic ulcers to reduce stomach acidity and relieve symptoms. Antibiotics may also be prescribed. Antibiotics, however, not only kill the bacteria causing the problem but the friendly bacteria as well, which can lead to other health problems.

Coconut oil offers another approach without harming the good bacteria. *H. pylori*, streptococcus, and herpes, which are all associated with various types of ulcers, are killed by the MCFAs in coconut oil. Coconut oil also possesses properties that fight cancer. Using coconut oil in the diet regularly is a safe and natural way to prevent and treat ulcers.

Bowel Disorders

Irritable bowel syndrome (IBS) affects the large intestine (colon). It is the most common disorder of the intestine, accounting for more than half the patients seen by gastroenterologists. After eating, IBS patients usually experience a combination of bloating, gas, abdominal pain, constipation, or diarrhea. These problems trigger an immune response causing flu-like symptoms—headaches, joint pain, muscle aches, and chronic fatigue.

Inflammatory bowel disease (IBD), not to be confused with IBS, includes, Crohn's disease, and ulcerative colitis. IBD is characterized by inflammation in the small or large intestine and may also include ulcers and tumorous growths. Symptoms include indigestion, nausea, abdominal pain, gas, diarrhea, and constipation. The incidence of IBD and IBS have greatly increased over the past 40 years and are far more common in developed countries where refined carbohydrates and medications are more frequently used.

Crohn's disease can affect any part of the gastrointestinal tract from the mouth to the rectum. The most common site of inflammation is the bottom portion of the small intestine where it joins the large intestine. Fever, bleeding, and weight loss may accompany it. Diarrhea can be almost continuous resulting in poor absorption of nutrients and loss of fluids and minerals. The intestinal wall becomes extremely thick due to continued chronic inflammation and deep, penetrating ulcers. The disease may affect other parts of the body such as the eyes and contribute to the development of skin disorders and arthritis.

Ulcerative colitis is chronic inflammation and ulceration of the lining of the colon and rectum. The main symptom is bloody diarrhea; the feces may also contain pus and mucus. In severe cases, diarrhea and bleeding can be extensive; fever may be present along with a general feeling of ill health. The loss of blood may lead to anemia. Other symptoms commonly associated with it include skin rashes, mouth ulcers, arthritis, and inflammation of the eyes. For those who have been affected for more than 10 years there is an increased risk of colon cancer. As with peptic ulcers the cause may be due to microorganisms, which cause chronic low-grade, localized infections and fever. As yet researchers have not identified any one particular bacterium or virus as the cause because the microorganisms that are creating the problem are normal inhabitants of the intestinal tract and their presence is not unexpected. Researchers are now beginning to recognize that overgrowth of the wrong types of bacteria may be the primary factor in inflammatory bowel disorders.[43]

Antibiotics have been used to treat inflammatory bowel disorders. Patients often experience relief from symptoms, but relief is generally short lived. When antibiotics are used, both the good and the bad bacteria are killed off, leaving yeast to multiply uninhibited and creating a new set of symptoms which antibiotics can't help. If dietary modifications and antibiotics don't bring lasting relief, surgery is the next option. Surgery, however, isn't a sure cure. Even after the infected segments of the intestine are removed, the condition often returns, infecting another part of the digestive tract. This is understandable because surgery doesn't correct the problem. The environment in the digestive tract is still out of balance.

A more sensible approach would be to improve intestinal health. Get it back into balance. This can be done by reducing sweets and refined grains, avoiding drugs that kill friendly bacteria, and eating foods which supply more fiber (vegetables, whole grains, coconut), by eating fermented foods (yogurt, kefir, and cultured coconut milk and water) that supply friendly bacteria, and using coconut oil which kills the disease causing bacteria and yeasts but not the friendly bacteria. Studies have shown that MCFAs are effective in reducing injury in the intestinal tract of animals when they are administered potent toxins. Inflammation is reduced and the immune response along the intestinal wall is enhanced.[44] So coconut oil can help protect and heal inflamed tissues along the digestive tract. People have reported that eating just two coconut macaroon cookies a day brings relief from symptoms associated with inflammatory bowel disease. Permanent relief, however, requires a little more effort.

Coconut oil can work wonders at helping to balance your intestinal environment; simply adding coconut products to your diet may be all you need. For some people with chronic inflammatory bowel disease a more aggressive approach may be in order. Let me illustrate. R.B. was a conventionally trained medical doctor. As a physician who believed in the use of medications to treat disease, he often used them himself to fight off infections and seasonal illnesses. These drugs, no doubt, took a toll on his health and he developed a severe case of inflammatory bowel disease accompanied by abdominal pain, constipation, and chronic fatigue. He spent 2½ years trying to overcome this problem and even turned to alternative medicine to find a solution. In desperation he went on a 30-day fast consuming nothing but water and dietary supplements. At the end of 30 days he felt only minor relief from his symptoms. Discouraged and searching, he ran across information about coconut oil and its affect on intestinal health. Still fasting, he added 15 tablespoons of coconut oil a day to his regimen. After 7 days with nothing but coconut oil, water, and vitamins, his symptoms completely disappeared. He felt better than he had in years. With the help of coconut oil this physician got his life back.

Gallbladder Disease

If you have gallbladder disease or have had your gallbladder surgically removed, you will find coconut oil a blessing. With coconut oil you will be able to add fat back into your diet without fear.

The gallbladder sits alongside and underneath the liver. It acts as a storage tank for bile, which is continuously being manufactured by the liver. When fat enters the intestinal tract a message is sent that signals the gallbladder to contract. As it does, bile is squirted down the bile duct into the intestine.

Bile is essential for fat digestion. Fat and water don't mix. When you combine water and oil, the oil floats to the surface. If you've ever made water and oil salad dressing this separation becomes very evident. The same thing happens in our digestive tract. Most of the food we eat is water-soluble and will separate from the fat. Fat digesting enzymes, which are water soluble, cannot mix with the oil. When bile is added it acts as an emulsifier, allowing the water and fat to mix. Fat digesting enzymes are then able to come into contact with all the fat molecules (triglycerides) and break them down into fatty acids.

The liver is continuously manufacturing bile. The small stream of bile being produced by the liver isn't adequate enough to handle a fatty meal. Therefore, the gallbladder is necessary in order to collect a large enough amount of bile to adequately handle the job.

A problem arises when bile in the gallbladder starts to solidify and develop into gallstones. Gallstones can reduce the amount of bile released into the intestines and even clog bile ducts, causing great pain and discomfort.

The standard solution to gallstones is to surgically remove the gallbladder. Another solution is to try to dissolve the stones with the use of ultrasound. Sound waves projected into the gallbladder break up the stones so that they flow out without clogging the bile ducts. If the stones are small this method may work. Unfortunately, by the time a person is aware that stones are present, the stones are too large for ultrasound to be effective.

A new approach to gallbladder disease is to use coconut oil in the diet. The monoglycerides and diglycerides of caprylic (C8) and capric (C10) acids in coconut oil have been found to dissolve gallstones in humans. The safe and efficient manner in which this is accomplished has been demonstrated at the Mayo Clinic and the University of Wisconsin Hospital.[45]

A major problem for people who have had gallbladder surgery is the inability to digest fat. Without a gallbladder there isn't enough bile present to adequately emulsify even a moderate amount of fat. Eat too much fat, and digestive distress becomes manifest. The discomfort is only a minor problem. The main concern is the lack of nutrition that results. An adequate amount of fat is necessary in the diet in order to get all the nutrients we need. Fat-soluble vitamins such as vitamins A, D, E, and K as well as beta-carotene require dietary fat for their absorption. If you don't digest fat, you won't get an adequate amount of these important vitamins. You can suffer from subclinical malnutrition, a vitamin and mineral deficiency that keeps you on the edge between enjoying good health and suffering from degenerative disease and illness. Although clearly defined symptoms of nutritional deficiencies are not necessarily manifest, health suffers, the immune system is depressed, aging is accelerated, and aches and pains slowly develop.

Adding more fat into the diet only causes intestinal distress. However, if you use coconut oil in place of other fats you can get the fat-soluble vitamins you need without the pain. As described earlier, MCTs in coconut oil digest very easily. Neither pancreatic digestive enzymes nor bile are necessary for their digestion. Therefore, coconut oil doesn't need as much bile for digestion as other fats do. People have reported that even though a small amount of fat can give them intestinal distress, they can eat two or more tablespoons of coconut at a time without problem. If you have had your gallbladder removed, try using coconut oil in place of other oils in your diet. Since everyone is different—some people are more sensitive to fats than others—go slow. Try a small amount at first and use only as much as you feel comfortable with.

FREE RADICALS AND ANTIOXIDANTS
The Link Between Free Radicals and Disease
What do all of the following conditions have in common: heart disease, cancer, hypertension, wrinkled skin, aging spots, arthritis, cataracts, and failing memory? You might say that all of these conditions are associated with aging, but age is not the cause. Indeed, even young people suffer from some of these ills. The one thing that ties all these conditions together, as well as most other degenerative diseases, is free radicals.

Free radicals are renegade molecular entities that cause destruction throughout the body. Free radicals are unstable molecules that have lost an electron, causing them to become highly reactive. In an effort to achieve equilibrium, they steal electrons from neighboring molecules. In the process, these other molecules themselves become free radicals, which in turn attack nearby molecules stealing their electrons. A chain reaction occurs where hundreds and even thousands of molecules are affected.

Once a molecule becomes a free radical, its physical and chemical properties change. The normal function of such molecules is permanently disrupted, affecting the entire cell of which they are a part. A living cell attacked by free radicals degenerates and becomes dysfunctional. Free radicals can attack our cells, literally ripping their protective membranes apart. Sensitive cellular components like the nucleus and DNA, which carries the genetic blueprint of the cell, can be damaged, leading to cellular mutations and death.

Free-radical damage has been linked to the loss of tissue integrity and to physical degeneration. As cells are bombarded by free radicals the tissues become progressively impaired. It is the accumulation of this damage over many years that result in the degeneration and loss of function that typifies the symptoms of old age. In fact, some researchers believe that free radicals are the primary cause of aging.

If free radicals were prevented from occurring inside our bodies, according to this theory, we would not age. Stopping free-radical reactions, however, is not possible. Free radicals are generated as a part of normal cellular respiration. Pollutants and toxins in our environment also cause them. Even our foods promote free-radical generation.

Free radicals are a product of oxidation. When iron oxidizes, free radicals are formed and rust develops. When fats oxidize, they become rancid. When tissues in the arteries oxidize, plaque is formed. Free radicals are destructive. If left unchecked they would damage every cell in the body. Fortunately, we have a means of self-protection. Our bodies produce many antioxidant enzymes that can stop free-radical chain reactions. Many nutrients in our foods such as vitamins C and E also act as antioxidants. The antioxidants in our bodies, and consequently the number of free radicals we have roaming around inside of us, depend on the types of foods we eat and our environment. If we live in a polluted environment and eat foods lacking in antioxidant nutrients, then free-radical destruction is severe. We age prematurely and develop any number of nagging chronic symptoms of degeneration.

Free radicals have been identified as the primary cause or at least a contributing factor to over 60 common health problems (see table on following page). Free radicals don't necessarily cause all of these conditions, but they are involved at least as accomplices. It has been suggested that most of the damage caused by these health problems is actually the result of free-radical destruction and not from the disease itself.

The Protective Role of Antioxidants and Coconut Oil

The oxidative process that occurs in fats is called *peroxidation*. Peroxidation is of major concern because it generates massive amounts of destructive free radicals that can have a significant impact on health. Unsaturated fats, particularly polyunsaturated fats, are highly prone to peroxidation and free-radical generation. Peroxidation of fats and oils can occur both in and outside of the body.

Scientists know that peroxidation in our bodies is involved in the development of many forms of cancers. Antioxidants have been found to be useful in protecting polyunsaturated fats from peroxidation, thus preventing

DISEASE AND FREE RADICALS

Some of the most common conditions involving free radicals.

Heart disease	Asthma
Atherosclerosis	Hay fever
Cancer	Food allergies
Stroke	Phlebitis
Diabetes	Ulcers
Psoriasis	Cataract
Eczema	Colitis
Acne	Constipation
Arthritis	Fibrocystic breast disease
Edema	Macular degeneration
Chronic fatigue	Alzheimer's disease
Varicose veins	Parkinson's disease
Hemorrhoids	Failing memory
Seizures	Senility
Prostitis	Kidney stones
Prostate hypertrophy	Gout
Multiple sclerosis	Depression
PMS	Insomnia
Dysmenorrhea	Lupus

the development of cancer. In one study, for instance, melanoma (skin cancer) cells treated with the antioxidant vitamin E showed significant decrease in cell proliferation, accompanied by a significant decrease of free-radical levels and lipid peroxidation.[46]

Antioxidants don't necessarily need to be taken orally to be effective. Topical applications of antioxidants have been shown to be effective in reducing risk of tumors in test animals.[47]

Karen Burke, M.D., Ph.D. of the Cabrini Medical Center in New York City reported that 240 skin cancer patients demonstrated significantly lower blood selenium (an antioxidant mineral) concentrations than control volunteers without skin cancer. To determine the protective quality of selenium, she ran tests on several groups of mice. One group was fed a selenium supplement, in another group a selenium compound was applied to the skin, and a third group received no treatment. All the groups were then subjected to ultraviolet radiation. Both treated groups showed far less damage than those that were not given selenium. Also, none of the animals given either oral or topical selenium developed any blistering sunburn, but the non-treated animals did.

This showed that selenium protected the fatty acids in the skin from UV radiation and reduced risk of skin cancer.[48, 49] This study also illustrates that protection from the effects of UV radiation can be obtained by both oral and topical application of an antioxidant.

Scientists discovered that chlorophyll could undergo free-radical formation within plant tissues. Carotenoids, a group of plant pigments that act as antioxidants, were found to protect against free-radical damage. Beta-carotene is the most well-known carotenoid. When researchers gave animals extra beta-carotene, they discovered that it also had a major protective effect against free radicals.[50] In human volunteers carotenoids protected the skin against the harmful effects of ultraviolet radiation. Volunteers significantly reduced their erythema (skin reddening) upon exposure to UV radiation after taking a supplement of mixed carotenoids.[51]

From studies like those above we know antioxidants are effective in protecting us from the cancer causing effects of free radicals. Coconut oil has the opposite effect of polyunsaturated fats. Numerous studies have shown that polyunsaturated oils promote cancer because they generate large amounts of free radicals that attack the DNA of our cells.[52] Because coconut oil functions as a protective antioxidant and decreases peroxidation, it should be helpful in protecting against cancer. Saturated fats are very stable chemically and are highly resistant to peroxidation and rancidity. This is why food manufactures like to add saturated fats to their products. Saturated fats help protect polyunsaturated fats from going rancid. The higher the saturated fatty acid content of a fat or oil the more stable it is and the more effective it is as an antioxidant. Coconut oil consists of 92 percent saturated fatty acids, which is higher than any other dietary fat. This makes it extremely stable and a valuable antioxidant. As an antioxidant, it helps protect against peroxidation of unsaturated fats and all the damage they cause.

Several recent studies have shown that polyunsaturated fat consumption is linked to macular degeneration.[53-55] Thirty years ago diabetes was the major cause of blindness and it was rare to find macular degeneration. Today the condition has overtaken diabetes five-fold and is now the leading cause of vision loss. In the United States two-thirds of those who lose their vision are blind due to macular degeneration. The belief over the past three decades that polyunsaturated vegetable oils were heart healthy has led to an increased use of these oils in place of other fats including coconut oil. Research shows that people who eat polyunsaturated vegetable oils get the disease twice as commonly as those who don't. Even more convincing was a study where they looked at patients with macular degeneration; the problem in those subjects who ate a lot of vegetable oil progressed at 3.8 times the rate of those eating only a little vegetable oil. Even monounsaturated oil was shown to increase risk. The lowest risk was associated with saturated fat, and the higher the saturation the better. Since coconut oil is the most highly saturated of all the dietary fats, it provides the greatest protection from macular degeneration. The problem with vegetable oils is that they create free radicals that damage the delicate tissues in the retina of the eye. Coconut oil, acting as an antioxidant, protects the eye from this damage.

Studies have shown that free radicals are involved in the occurrence of epileptic seizures. Coconut oil can be of benefit here as well. When added to the diet, MCFAs have proven to be effective in reducing epileptic seizures in children. D.L. Ross of the University of Minnesota Medical School found that seizure frequency decreased by more than 50 percent in two-thirds of the epileptic children in his study during a 10-week treatment period.[56]

One of the primary causes of dry, wrinkled skin associated with aging is free-radical damage. Dry skin is associated with unsaturated fatty acids. In one study it was found dry skin contained a higher content of unsaturated fatty acids (60 percent) than normal skin (49 percent).[57] Discoloration of the skin, such as liver spots, is also a sign of free-radical destruction. We can see the effects of free-radical destruction on the skin, but the same process occurs inside the body as well. If your body is aging on the outside, it's also aging on the inside. The more unsaturated fat in the skin, the greater the degree of free-radical damage and the greater the risk of premature aging, wrinkles, discolorations, and cancer.

Reducing the amount of free-radical damage you experience will keep you looking and feeling younger as you grow older. Regular consumption of coconut oil will help keep free radicals at bay and slow down the aging process.

Coconut oil use can affect the health of the entire body and can be useful in preventing "dis-ease." Dis-ease being defined as any form of discomfort caused by degeneration, sickness, or feelings of ill health that put the body or mind at dis-ease. Free radicals can cause a lot of dis-ease.

Because coconut oil acts as a protective antioxidant it can conceivably help prevent or at least reduce some of the symptoms associated with the many health problems linked to free radicals.

CANCER

When I was first beginning to use coconut oil and telling others about it, one of the things I noticed is that when it was applied topically it would clear up a number of skin problems. The skin of people with hard crusty growths, scabs, and moles became smooth and soft. Even precancerous lesions vanished with regular use. One man had several hardened, precancerous lesions on his scalp. The lesions were somewhat tender, slightly inflamed, and never healed. Since they were on his scalp and essentially out of sight he ignored them. He thought they were minor sores and paid no attention. They persisted for three or four years before he became concerned. I had him put coconut oil on the lesions, following the procedure recommended by Paul Sorse (see Chapter 1). Within a month the lesions had completely healed. I've seen similar results in others. Pet owners are seeing results too. One pet owner who makes her own dog food (kibble) using coconut oil states, "I use it in making the kibble, and on it just before I give it to them. I have noticed a remarkable difference in their health, as seen in their eyes, energy levels, coats, etc. The two males had recently been diagnosed with cancer, and now they are cancer free...My holistic vet reports that he has never seen cancer gone so quickly! By the way, that same vet is now a believer in coconut oil and he regularly prescribes it for all of his patients." From incidences like these it is apparent that coconut oil possesses anticancer properties. Medical research backs this up. Several studies show the anticancer effects of coconut oil particularly in association with colon, breast, and skin cancers and possibly liver cancer as well.

In one study, for example, colon cancer was chemically induced in a group of rats.[58] The animals were fed diets containing different types of fat to determine their influence on cancer. Oils tested included corn, safflower, olive, fractionated coconut, and coconut oils. Coconut oil inhibited the development of cancer more than any of the fats tested. In the colon (large intestine) there

MY BATTLE WITH CANCER

In 1998, I was running a computer company in New York. I also had an Internet company in the Philippines and was in charge of a very exciting Internet trade show in Asia (Internet World). I was very busy and enjoying work but always made sure I got my yearly executive check up, including my yearly mammogram. In February of 1998 I got a clean bill of health.

A few months later I began feeling a strange sensation in by breasts. By late October it developed into a sharp pain. I went to the doctor and was immediately referred to an oncologist for testing. I was told I had a very aggressive form of breast cancer and needed surgery immediately.

This came as a shock to me. I began to wonder why? There was no history of cancer in my family. Was it the toxic waste in New Jersey where I had lived for the past ten years? Was I stressed at work and did not know it? I thought there had to be a reason why people get cancer.

Before going through with a mastectomy I wanted a second opinion. I went to a different specialist but he told me the same thing. I kept trying to find a doctor that would tell me that all I needed was a lumpectomy or just chemotherapy. Finally, the fifth doctor told it to me straight, "You don't have a choice. We don't even know if we can still save you. You are at stage 4, the most serious stage, we need to do the surgery immediately."

Here I was, in February cancer free, now just eight months later I was knocking on death's door with a very aggressive form of breast cancer. I went through with the operation and afterwards several months of chemotherapy. While doctors said that the cancer was under control, it wasn't completely gone. So they kept me on medication.

I decided to go back to the Philippines for a visit. I owned a farm there that I loved and had always wanted to grow medicinal plants. The farm was filled with coconut trees, which were harvested for the copra. I thought about planting coffee under the coconut trees and start an herbal medicine garden.

Then in 2001 I began to experience painful headaches. They became so severe that it felt like the bones in my skull were being fractured. I walked into my doctor's office and told him I wanted an X-ray of my skull. "Were you in an accident" he questioned?

"No" I said, "I just feel that I have some kind of fracture in my skull."

He smiled, "How do you know you have a fracture? Maybe a stronger pain killer will solve your problem."

"I know what a fracture feels like." I said, "I've had several bones broken in the past and I know what it feels like."

He didn't argue any further and I had an X-ray taken. I went back the next day to see my doctor and instead, met with seven other doctors. They had never seen the type of skull cancer I had. Almost half my skull looked like cheese that had been eaten by rats. I was in shock. I asked them what were

my chances for survival? They said, "In the Philippines, at your stage...none."
I probably had two months.

I took the next flight to the United States. I went to see my doctor the afternoon I arrived. The doctors in Manila had already faxed and spoken to him about my condition. The next day I visited with my neurosurgeon. We discussed my condition and scheduled a craniotomy. My prognosis was poor. He ordered an MRI, CT scans, bone scans, blood work, etc. This was the same cancer that had so aggressively attacked me before. It had now spread up into my skull. Surgery was scheduled for the morning after.

The cancer was hairline close to the main artery in my brain. The bad news was that he could not take it all out; 20% of it was at the back of my skull in the center over the main artery. Chemotherapy had not been successful after breast surgery so there was little hope it would be of any use now. But at this point, it was the only hope I had.

My chances for survival were grim. I knew I'd better make the most of the time I had remaining. After several months of recovery from the surgery I went back to my farm in Philippines to visit my family.

I was really weak and would just sit on the hill watching the farmers work among the coconut trees planting coffee seedlings. I knew I had to do something to strengthen my immune system. I wanted to plant an herb garden. I started doing research on what medicinal plants I should grow that would boost my immune system. I thought about planting ginseng or bitter melons. I even considered growing a shrub from the Amazon.

Just about that time, I came across some research on coconut oil. I read about clinical trials for AIDS in the Philippines using coconut oil. I figured if coconut oil can boost the immune system and cure AIDS, it might work for my cancer.

I started taking 3 to 4 tablespoons of oil a day plus whatever I used in preparing my meals. I would add it to my oatmeal in the morning, put it in my hot chocolate, cook my meals in it. I also snacked on fresh coconut and drank coconut juice.

By July my doctors started to worry. I had been gone for nearly six months. They needed to monitor the cancer that was still in my skull. So I flew back to the US. To their complete surprise I had gone into remission. They asked me what I had done. I told them I found a cure—virgin coconut oil. Today I continue to use coconut oil and I am cancer free!

I had grown up around coconut trees in the Philippines. My grandmother used to make coconut oil from fresh coconuts just as many of the farmers did. I never used it because we were told it was a saturated fat. We were health conscious so we used hydrogenated soybean oil and corn oil. I had coconut oil around me all my life. It took getting cancer and a desperate search for a cure that made me rediscover this miracle oil.

Julie Figueroa

was a 10-fold difference in tumor development between those that received corn oil and those that received coconut oil. Rats fed coconut oil and olive oil had the lowest incidence of tumors occurring in the small intestine. Olive oil had 7 percent while the coconut oil fed animals had none.

The anticancer effects of MCFAs in coconut oil have also been demonstrated with chemically induced breast cancer.[59] Studies by L.A. Cohen and colleagues found that the animals given MCFAs in their diet did not develop tumors while those fed other oils did. Cohen stated that there were no detectable tumor-promoting effects in the MCFA-fed animals even though they were administered potent mammary cancer-causing chemicals.[60]

Coconut oil can protect the skin from cancer as well. When cancer-causing chemicals were applied on the skin of mice, tumors developed within 20 weeks. However, when coconut oil was applied along with the chemicals, there was a complete absence of tumor development. [61]

Stored grains and legumes are frequently contaminated with aflatoxin, a cancer-causing substance produced by mold. Aflatoxin is known to cause liver cancer in animals and is believed to be responsible for the high incidence of liver cancer in Africa and Asia. Liver cancer is a serious problem in some parts of the Philippines. Corn has been found to be the most aflatoxin contaminated food eaten in the Philippines. In certain areas of the country corn consumption is high. A correlation exists between the incidence of liver cancer and the amount of corn consumed. Those people who eat the most corn also have the highest rates of liver cancer. Coconut oil consumption appears to protect the liver from the cancer-causing effect of aflatoxin.[62] The population of Bicol has an unusually high intake of coconut as well as a high intake of corn. The coconut apparently protects them from the effects of aflatoxin because they have a much lower incidence of liver cancer than in other parts of the Philippines.

The anti-cancer effects of the MCTs in coconut oil were demonstrated in yet another study. MCT oil (which contains 100 percent MCTs) was combined with fish oil and fed to rats with chemically induced sarcoma. Sarcoma is cancer of the connective or fibrous tissues that surround and supports organs. This study revealed that MCT/fish oil feeding inhibited tumor growth, which was attributed to a decrease in tumor protein syntheses.[63]

Cancer can be caused by a number of factors such as free radicals and carcinogenic chemicals, the effects of which appear to be tempered by coconut oil. Another known cause of cancer is viruses. Human papillomavirus (HPV), for instance, is found in virtually every case of cervical cancer. Other viruses that may be linked to cancer include Epstein-Barr virus, cytomegalovirus, and adenovirus. Coconut may be helpful in preventing these cancers because of MCFAs anti-viral effects. In this way coconut oil provides another means of protection against cancer.

Every single one of us has cancerous cells in our bodies. The reason we don't all develop cancer and die is because the immune system destroys these renegade cells before they can get out of hand. As long as the immune system is functioning in the manner for which it was designed, we need not worry about cancer. Arthur I. Holleb, M.D., senior vice president of Medical Affairs for the American Cancer Society states: "Only when the immune system is incapable of destroying these malignant cells will cancer develop."[64] In other words, cancer can only develop in those individuals whose immune systems are so stressed or weakened that they are incapable of mounting an effective defense. Dr. Holleb doesn't specify that the efficiency of the immune system affects only lung cancer or breast cancer or leukemia. He refers to all cancers, which means that even if we are exposed to carcinogenic substances, if the immune system is working as it should, cancer will not develop. A healthy immune system, therefore, is a key element in the prevention of all forms of cancer.

Because coconut oil protects against cancer, some researchers believe that medium-chain fatty acids enhance the immune system. Witcher and associates tested this hypothesis and found that that monolaurin, a monoglyceride of lauric acid, stimulates the production of white blood cells, specifically T cells. T cells attack and kill anything that is foreign to the body including cancerous cells. T cells play a significant role in our defense against cancer.[65]

Another study shows that MCFAs can influence the fatty acid composition of tumor tissue and tumor protein kinetics inhibiting tumor growth.[66]

From the evidence we have so far, we know that coconut oil acts as a protective antioxidant that stops the destructive action and cancer-promoting effect of free radicals. It enhances the immune system, which actively fights these renegade cells. It appears to be able to block the uncontrolled growth of cancer cells. Coconut oil also protects cells against the mutagenic effects of carcinogens. Since there is no harm in using coconut oil, using it internally and externally may provide a safe and effective way to protect yourself from cancer.

LIVER DISEASE

As an antioxidant, coconut oil can provide protection not only from cancer but also from a variety of free-radical related health problems. For example, MCFAs in coconut oil have been shown to prevent the destructive action of free radicals in the liver. A study by H. Kono and colleagues showed that MCFAs can prevent alcohol-induced liver injury by inhibiting free-radical formation.[67] Several other studies have also shown that fatty acids, such as those found in coconut oil, protect the liver from alcohol-induced free-radical injury and tissue death, indicating that the use of coconut oil can not only prevent injury but even rejuvenate diseased tissue. Dr. A. Nanji and other researchers have recommended using fatty acids (from tropical oils) as a dietary treatment for alcoholic liver disease.[68, 69]

Of all the organs in the body, the liver probably receives the greatest benefit from coconut oil. The liver is under constant stress, filtering out waste, neutralizing toxins, dismantling and reconstructing fats and proteins, storing and producing energy, and performing a hundred other functions. Disease causing germs and damaging free radicals constantly attack the liver, affecting its function. MCFAs from coconut oil help relieve the stress by stopping free radicals and killing harmful germs. Coconut oil also functions as a natural detoxification agent by neutralizing the effects of poisons. Eating coconut oil gives the liver a break, reducing its workload, protecting it from free radicals, and supplying it with needed energy. Remember, MCFAs are used by the liver as a source of fuel to power and stimulate metabolism. MCTs appear to enhance liver function.[70]

Coconut oil also helps keep the liver from clogging up with cholesterol. Diets with MCFAs significantly lower levels of liver cholesterol compared to those consisting of LCFAs. This may sound contrary to what is commonly believed, but oils composed of LCFAs, such as soybean and canola, produce a significantly higher level of liver cholesterol than does coconut oil.[71]

Although the intake of unsaturated vegetable oils is associated with decreased blood cholesterol levels, they increase tissue cholesterol, including cholesterol in the liver. Consumption of polyunsaturated vegetable oil reduces blood cholesterol. But when cholesterol leaves the blood where does it go? It doesn't just magically disappear. What happens is that the cholesterol is pulled out of the blood and driven into the tissues. Although the blood may have a lower level of cholesterol the surrounding tissues will have a higher level. Eating too much vegetable oil composed of LCFAs can clog the liver with cholesterol. In contrast, MCFAs decrease the level of cholesterol in the liver. In fact MCFAs tends to reduce cholesterol in all tissues.[72]

A. B. Awad compared the effects of diets containing 14 percent coconut oil, 14 percent safflower oil or a 5 percent control (mostly soybean) oil on accumulation of cholesterol in tissues in rats. The synthetic diets had 2 percent added corn oil with a total fat of 16 percent. Total tissue cholesterol accumulation for animals on the safflower diet was six times greater than for animals fed the coconut oil, and twice that of the animals fed the low fat control diet.[73]

KIDNEY DISEASE

The kidneys perform many functions that are vital to health. Their primary function is to filter the blood and dispose of waste products. They also regulate electrolytes, pH, and blood pressure as well as maintain fluid balance. As we age, the efficiency of the kidneys diminishes. If kidney function decreases too much it can lead to kidney failure and death. So keeping your kidneys healthy helps keep you healthy.

Evidence suggests that coconut oil may help protect your kidneys from harm and keep them functioning properly. In one study, for example, where kidney failure was induced in test animals, those that were given coconut oil had fewer and less severe lesions and survived longer. The researchers concluded that coconut oil has a protective effect on the kidneys.[74]

Diabetic nephropathy is a form of kidney disease that occurs in diabetics. Kidney failure is one of the leading causes of death in diabetics. When blood sugar levels are not controlled over long periods of time circulatory problems can occur, causing damage to the small capillaries in the kidneys. I have seen diabetics with serious circulation problems gain relief from their symptoms after they began using coconut oil. If the damage is not too severe, recovery is possible. If permanent damage has already been done, the oil can keep the kidneys from getting worse.

Selina Sayong knows the benefits of coconut oil. In 1991 she suffered liver and kidney failure. She underwent dialysis for two years and had a transplant in 1994. In 2000 the new kidney was rejected. She began working with a new doctor who became interested in the healing properties of coconut oil. With her permission and knowing it wouldn't do her any harm, he used her as a guinea pig of sorts to test the benefits of the oil. She began noticing changes in just two weeks, starting with having regular bowel movements (dialysis patients suffer from constipation), to an overall feeling of being cleansed and detoxified. Although Selina still undergoes dialysis, she is full of life and energy. She has become so excited about her new lease on life that in addition to working full time as an advertising and marketing consultant, she started a new business selling coconut products. As if that wasn't enough to keep her busy, in her spare time she teaches motivational and wellness seminars. While the coconut oil couldn't reverse the permanent damage, it has given her the energy and motivation to live life to the fullest.

DETOXIFICATION

We are exposed to an endless variety of pollutants and toxins in the air we breathe, the foods we eat, and the water we drink. Harmful chemicals, both natural and man-made, as well as disease-causing germs are swarming around us 24 hours a day. No matter what we do, we cannot prevent contact with all harmful substances. Nor can we stop all toxins from entering our bodies. Fortunately, our bodies are capable of neutralizing and eliminating a great deal of these toxic substances to maintain good health.

However, when exposure to toxins is high, they can accumulate in the body faster than they can be eliminated. As these toxins build up, they slowly poison the body. The result is degeneration, premature aging, sickness, and chronic disease. Cancer is a perfect example of the consequences of toxic accumulation. As carcinogenic substances accumulate in the body they poison cells, causing them to become mutated or diseased. The result is cancer.

Toxic buildup can affect every part of the body and contribute to a wide variety of health problems ranging from asthma to yeast infections. Toxins also generate free radicals that further burden the body. As toxins and free radicals accumulate, the immune system becomes overburdened and less effective. The body becomes more susceptible to illness. Aches, pains, and chronic health problems develop. This is why a good detoxification program can greatly improve overall health and even reverse serious health problems.

One of the weapons of alternative medicine is detoxification. If toxins can be removed from the body the immune system will function more efficiently and health will improve. The improvement can be so dramatic that even chronic or serious health problems can be overcome.

There are many natural substances that can aid in cleansing excess toxins from the body. Coconut oil is one of these. One of the things I often hear from people who start adding coconut oil into their diet is that they experience cleaning reactions. Why does coconut oil have a cleansing effect? I can think of four reasons:

1. MCFAs in coconut oil kill disease-causing bacteria, viruses, fungi, and parasites. These microorganisms not only cause infection but also often produce toxic byproducts that are carcinogenic or poisonous.

2. Coconut oil is chemically very stable so it functions as an antioxidant protecting against destructive free radicals that are often generated by toxins.[75]

3. MCFAs in coconut oil are used by the body as a source of fuel to stimulate metabolism. As metabolism increases so does the body's natural mechanisms of detoxification, repair, and growth. Even the immune system is shifted to a higher level of efficiency.[76]

4. Coconut oil neutralizes the harmful effects of many toxins including the deadly aflatoxin.[77]

Because of coconut oil's antioxidant and anti-inflammatory properties and its ability to supply a quick source of cellular energy and improve oxygen utilization, it neutralizes or blocks the detrimental effects of many harmful chemicals. Studies show that when coconut oil is given to animals that are exposed to a variety of different carcinogenic chemicals they are protected from developing cancer.[78] Kono and associates have found that MCTs enhance the immune system and reduce inflammation when animals are administered toxins.[79]

Glutamic acid, a neurotoxin that affects the function of the brain and nerves, is tempered by monoglycerides from coconut oil.[80] Glutamic acid is the primary component of monosodium glutamate (MSG) which is a common food additive. In animals glutamic acid causes brain lesions and neuroendocrine disorders. In humans it can do the same. Some of the symptoms associated with it include seizures, stroke, and heart irregularities among others.[81]

Reddy and colleagues fed rats different types of fat. Colon cancer was induced in the animals with the chemical azoxymethane. The research team found that corn and safflower oils promoted the development of cancer while coconut oil prevented it.[82]

Similarly, Cohen and Thompson found that mammary cancer induced by the chemical N-nitrosomethylurea was promoted by corn oil but inhibited by a mixture of 75 percent coconut oil derived MCTs and 25 percent corn oil. It is interesting that corn oil promotes cancer yet the MCTs in the mixture negated this detrimental effect and still prevented the development of tumors in the test animals.[83]

Dr. C. Lim-Sylianco and colleagues demonstrated coconut oil's antimutagenic effects against six potent mutacarcinogens—benzpyrene, azaserine, dimethylhydrazine, dimethynitrosamine, methylmethanesulfonate, and tetracycline. Administration of coconut oil either in bolus doses or as part of the diet protected the animals from the toxic effect of all six mutagens. Fertility tests were also performed and coconut oil was shown to protect fertilized female mice against the sterilizing and abortifacient effects of the carcinogens. Dr. Lim-Sylianco reported that coconut oil was "strongly protective" against all six chemicals.[84, 85]

Studies have shown that the harmful effects of exotoxins and endotoxins— poisons produced by bacteria—can also be neutralized or reduced by the use of coconut oil and its monoglycerides. Monoglycerides of coconut oil are commonly used in the food and cosmetic industry to inhibit the production of exotoxins produced by streptococci and staphylococci.[86, 87] As a point of interest, in addition to neutralizing these poisons, MCFAs and their monoglycerides are potent antimicrobials that can kill both streptococci and staphylococci, another benefit against infectious disease.

Both monoglycerides and MCFAs in coconut oil neutralize the effects of these poisons inside the body. For example, in one study guinea pigs were separated into two groups. One group was given a mixture of MCTs and fish oil in their diet. The other group received safflower oil. After 6 weeks on this diet the animals were injected with an endotoxin. The group fed safflower oil developed severe metabolic and respiratory shock. The group that received MCTs showed only mild symptoms. [88]

In another study, the protective effect of coconut oil was tested on *E. coli* endotoxin shock in rats.[89] A total of 180 rats were used in the study. The animals were separated into three equal groups. The first group was given coconut oil at 5 percent of daily calories in their diet; the second group 20 percent; and the third received no coconut oil and served as the control. After one month on the diet the rats were given, by oral tube, a dose of *E. coli* endotoxin. The number of survivors was monitored at intervals of up to 96 hours. The results showed that rats in the control group had only a 48 percent survival rate. Those given coconut oil at 5 percent and 20 percent of total calories had survival rates of 77 percent and 72 percent, respectively. Both coconut oil fed groups had about the same level of survival. This indicated that even a small amount of coconut oil (5 percent of calories) offered the same amount of protection against *E coli* endotoxin as a larger amount (20 percent of calories). In humans consuming a typical 2,000-calorie diet, 5 percent of calories would equate to about 1 tablespoon of coconut oil.

Our environment is full of toxins. Air pollution is of major concern. Not only are we subjected to car exhaust and factory pollution, but even the air in our own homes can be toxic. Chemicals used in drapes, carpets, varnish, paint, glue, insecticides, and mold are common indoor pollutants. Indoor pollution can even be worse than the smog outside. When I moved from my old residence to a new house, I learned just how detrimental indoor pollution can be. The house was newly painted and carpeted. Stain and varnish was freshly applied to wood surfaces. The house smelled like a glue factory. After living in the house for a few days, I developed a chronic headache, dizziness, and constant fatigue. I felt terrible. During the move I had packed away my coconut oil so

Toxins Mitigated by Coconut Oil

Studies show that coconut oil tempers or blocks the harmful effects of many toxins including the following:

Ethanol	Dimethynitrosamine
Glutamic acid/MSG	Methylmethanesulfonate
N-nitrosomethylurea	Tetracycline
Azoxymethane	Streptococci endotoxin/exotoxin
Benzpyrene	Staphylococci endotoxin/exotoxin
Azaserine	E. coli endotoxin
Dimethylbenzanthracene	Aflatoxin
Dimethylhydrazine	

I hadn't had any for a couple of weeks. Realizing that my symptoms were due to the toxic fumes and knowing about coconut oil's detoxifying effect, I put a couple of tablespoons of oil in a cup of hot herbal tea. Within a couple of hours my head cleared up and my energy slowly started to return. By the next day I was feeling great. I made sure that I didn't neglect my daily dose of coconut oil after that.

Studies suggest that coconut oil can provide protection from a variety of natural and man-made toxins in our environment. My own personal experience seems to verify this. For this reason, it can be a valuable aid as a means of detoxification and cleansing. Using coconut oil regularly can help neutralize many of the harmful toxins we are exposed to each day. It can be a remarkable aid in detoxifying and cleansing the body. Experience has shown that detoxifying effects of coconut oil can be so potent that it may cause intense cleansing reactions in some individuals. This is discussed in more detail in Chapter 7.

THE SUNSHINE VITAMIN

We live in the dark, so to speak. Doctors tell us to avoid the sun at all costs because it causes skin cancer. Our fear of this dreaded disease has driven us out of the sun. We are taught to run for cover whenever the sun pokes its head up. We spend almost all of our time shielded indoors. When we do go outside we are encouraged to wear enough clothing to cover every patch of skin and plaster sunscreen on every exposed cell to protect us from the evil rays of the sun. UV radiation, we are told, will give us cancer. About 1 million cases of skin cancer are diagnosed annually in the United States. The most deadly form of skin cancer, melanoma, is diagnosed in about 55,000 Americans annually. Sounds frightening. No wonder we are afraid of the sun.

Believe it or not, UV radiation is actually *good* for you, at least in moderation. Although it can promote cancer if you get too much, at reasonable levels it will help protect against it. In fact, running away from sunlight *increases* your chances of getting cancer. Most cases of melanoma occur on the back and legs—areas that are typically protected from sunlight. The face, hands, and arms, which receive the most sun exposure are the least likely places to develop melanoma.

A study conducted by the US Navy compared the risk of melanoma for different naval occupations. It was discovered that those with indoor jobs had the *highest* incidence of melanoma, while those who worked at least part of the time outdoors had the lowest rate. In addition, a higher rate of melanoma occurred on the trunk of the body that was covered by clothing, as opposed to the head and arms, which are more likely to be exposed to sunlight. The authors of the study stated that the location of the melanomas suggest a *protective* role for regular exposure to sunlight.[90] Sunlight appears to offer protection not just from melanoma but from all types of cancer. Studies have shown that sunlight reduces the risk for at least 17 different types of cancer including breast, colon, rectal, lung, and prostate cancers.

Besides protecting us from cancer, sunlight has a great influence on other aspects of our health. One of the primary benefits of sunlight, and more specifically UV light, is the production of vitamin D. Vitamin D is often called the sunshine vitamin because it is made inside our bodies when UV light strikes our skin. Because of our fear of sunlight and skin cancer, it is estimated that up to 70 percent of all Americans have a vitamin D deficiency. This is serious because vitamin D influences our health in many ways.

For decades it has been known that vitamin D is essential in calcium metabolism and is necessary for proper bone growth and development. Without adequate vitamin D, bones become thin, soft, and misshapen. Children who suffer from a deficiency develop rickets. Bones fail to calcify normally and may become so weak that they become deformed by the body's weight. Bowed legs are characteristic of the disease. In adults the condition is called osteomalacia. Signs are pain in the pelvis, lower back, legs, and susceptibility to fractures. Osteoporosis and low back pain that are so common in our society nowadays may be warning signs of a vitamin D deficiency.

In recent years medical research has been identifying many additional health problems associated with vitamin D deficiency. These include:

Cancer
Heart disease
Hypertension
Multiple sclerosis (MS)
Diabetes
Osteoporosis
Arthritis
Muscle and back pain
Inflammatory bowel disease
Psoriasis
Autoimmune illnesses

These are not just casual relationships. Studies show, for example, that vitamin D can reduce colon cancer and type 1 diabetes risk by 80 percent and cut MS by 40 percent. This is significant. Simply getting more sunlight and more UV rays can reduce your chances of getting these conditions and help to improve or totally eliminate symptoms if they are already present.

Vitamin D is one of the main reasons why sunlight provides protection against cancer. It moderates cell growth and slows down hyperactive cell proliferation, thus helping to keep cancer in check.[91] Vitamin D deficiency is also associated with insulin deficiency and insulin resistance.[92-94] It is a major factor in the development of type I diabetes in children.[95] Because a deficiency promotes insulin resistance, it may also be a factor in type II diabetes as well. Insulin resistance, hypertension, and chronic inflammation are all major risk factors for heart disease, and each can be caused by a vitamin D deficiency. I feel that you can get a far greater degree of protection from heart disease simply by getting regular exposure to the sun than you can by monitoring your cholesterol levels and taking cholesterol-lowering drugs. And sunshine doesn't cost you a dime.

Dietary sources of vitamin D include eggs, fish, organ meats, and animal fat. Vitamin D is stored in the fat of animals that are exposed to the sun. With the exception of fatty fish, cod liver oil, and lard, the amount of vitamin D in foods is very small and it would be difficult to get an adequate amount just from dietary sources. Sunlight is essential. You can get all of the vitamin D you need from the sun. Actually, that's the best source.

The optimal time to get sunlight is between 10:00 am and 4:00 pm. This is the time when UV light, which stimulates the production of vitamin D, is at its greatest intensity. Any exposure earlier or later drastically reduces UV light exposure. UV light is filtered through the atmosphere. The more atmosphere through which UV light travels, the weaker it gets. In early morning and late afternoon so little UV light reaches the earth that essentially no vitamin D is formed.

Likewise, in winter the sun can be at an angle so that little UV light reaches the earth's surface. Below a latitude of 35 degrees (0 degrees is at the equator), the angle of the sun is such that vitamin D synthesis can occur in the skin year-round. However, above 35 degrees the angle of the sun is so oblique during the winter months that most, if not all, of the UV light is absorbed in the atmosphere, reducing or completely preventing the production of vitamin D in the skin. For example, residents of Boston (42 degrees N), Edmonton, Canada (52 degrees N), and Helsinki, Finland (61 degrees N) cannot produce sufficient quantities of vitamin D in their skin for 4, 5, and 6 months, respectively.

The general recommendation of 20 minutes a day of direct sunlight on the face and arms is sufficient to produce 200 to 400 IU of vitamin D, which satisfies the recommended daily allowance (RDA). This is enough to prevent rickets, but it is not enough to prevent many of the other conditions associated with vitamin D deficiency. Researchers are now recommending that we get at least 1,000 IU and as much as 2,000 IU a day.

To get 1,000-2,000 IU a day would require 30-60 minutes or more in the sun with as much flesh exposed as possible. The time you need would vary depending on time of day, time of year, latitude, altitude, and weather. The best time is at mid-day as noted above. You need more exposure in winter than in summer. The higher in elevation you are, the greater the intensity of the sun and the more UV light you receive. Clouds will block out the UV rays. You need direct sunlight outdoors. Sitting in a sunny spot indoors doesn't work. UV light, which is essential for vitamin D synthesis, is filtered out as it passes through glass.

You can supplement what you get from the sun with food or dietary supplements. Cod liver oil is one of the richest sources of vitamin D.

You don't need to worry about getting too much vitamin D from the sun. Sunbathers can get all the sunlight they need within 20-30 minutes. Our bodies have a self-regulating system that limits the amount it makes, which is 20,000 IU. This is more than the body needs in a day but the excess is stored for rainy days. You can get this amount with full-sun exposure over the entire body during the summer within an hour or two. In the winter it may be impossible to get even the daily amount needed no matter how long you are in the sun. Dark-skinned people make less vitamin D. They may need three hours of sun exposure to get the same effect as a light-skinned person gets in 30 minutes.

Getting too much sun will not hurt you so long as you don't get sunburned or become overly red. Sunburns damage the skin and promote cancer so you want to avoid excessive exposure. Unfortunately, it is not easy to tell when you have had enough until it is too late. Sunscreen isn't the answer. Sunscreens with a protection factor of as little as 8 block about 94 percent of the UV rays and thus prevent vitamin D synthesis. Some studies show that the chemicals in these creams may promote cancer, so they could do more harm than good.

A far better option to sunscreen would be to use coconut oil. Applied on the skin it protects against sunburn as well as cancer. Unlike sunscreen, coconut oil does not block the UV rays that are necessary for vitamin D synthesis. It protects the skin and underlying tissues from damage excessive exposure can cause. Instead of burning or turning red it produces a light tan, depending on the length of time you spend in the sun. Consuming coconut oil also strengthens the skin and makes it more resilient and less prone to sunburn.

The types of fats we eat affect how our bodies respond to sunlight. Fats in the diet are incorporated into skin tissues. Polyunsaturated fats are easily oxidized by sunlight, causing destructive free-radical reactions that initiate the cancer process. People who eat a lot of polyunsaturated oils are more vulnerable to sunburn and skin cancer.

Assimilation and utilization of vitamin D is also affected by dietary fat intake. Both polyunsaturated and monounsaturated fats in the diet decrease the binding of vitamin D to D-binding proteins and thus make the vitamin less available for utilization in the body.[96] Unsaturated fats like soybean and canola oils actually promote vitamin D deficiency. Saturated fats, such as coconut oil, do not have this effect. So if you are going to get the most benefit from sunbathing, coconut oil should be the main source of fat in your diet.

BRAIN HEALTH

"Rita is my Miracle Lady," says her husband Edwin Vaughn. "For many years she suffered with Alzheimer's and diabetes, both of which are now gone for the most part, or on the way out, thanks to coconut oil. I could exclaim about coconut oil from the mountain tops, it is so super! Our family had mostly given up on her when our doctor suggested that we try giving her coconut oil. After she began taking coconut oil I can't believe the miracle that have happened, that's why I call her my Miracle Lady.

"In just a few weeks, things started to change for the better. Rita was getting insulin twice a day—every morning and afternoon. Then with taking coconut oil in her yogurt two or three times a day, her blood sugar went to normal! Her morning insulin was completely stopped and only occasionally did she take it in the afternoon. As for Rita's Alzheimer's, her mind and memory are wonderfully improved! The disease has reversed.

"One nice thing about my beautiful wife is that she has returned to making people laugh and feel better. She has always loved to talk, but for the past couple of years she hardly ever spoke. When she tried to say something the words and sentences came out garbled and we couldn't understand her, so she stopped communicating for the most part. After taking coconut oil, her speech has dramatically improved; she now speaks in clear sentences and is easy to understand. She smiles a lot and has become her old talkative self again. As her many friends know, she loves to talk and laugh. The folks at the Meals on Wheels and the senior center know that she would rather talk than eat. Rita still does both, and amazingly, too."

Few other diseases can elicit the fear and sense of hopelessness that comes with a diagnosis of Alzheimer's. Ever since it was first identified by Dr. Alois Alzheimer in 1906 there has been little hope for those who have the disease.

The gradual decline in mental function associated with Alzheimer's often begins with barely noticeable lapses in memory followed by losses in the ability to plan and execute familiar tasks, and to reason and execute judgment. Eventually, memory loss increases in severity until it is incapacitating. The ability to articulate words correctly and changes in mood and personality may also be evident. Emotional problems such as easy agitation, poor judgment, mental confusion, feelings of withdrawal, disorientation, and hallucinations are common. Affected individuals may also develop seizures and incontinence, requiring constant attention and care. Death is the final outcome.

Alzheimer's Disease

My mother has Alzheimer's disease. Eventually, we moved her to a nearby nursing home. When she got there she was doing things like sleeping at the dinner table, not communicating well except to answer questions with simple answers like "Yes" and 'No", etc. I started her on a few tablespoons of coconut oil per day. Within a few weeks she began being more easily engaged in conversation, laughing more, and not sleeping at much. A nurse, a physical therapist, and a speech therapist pulled me aside (on different days) and asked if I'd been doing anything different with mom. When I told them that I'd been adding coconut oil to her food daily, their mouths dropped open.

Audley L.

Parkinson's Disease

I currently care for my 85-year-old father who has a multitude of problems, including dementia, Parkinson's symptoms, and lymphatic cancer. He definitely had all the signs of Parkinson's, but the doctors would not diagnose him with the Parkinson's as he was having the symptoms prior to our getting him to go to the doctor. When I told the doctor that he had been shaking, shuffling gait, flat-faced affect, stooped over walking and it had cleared up with virgin coconut oil, he just looked at me and said that it could not have been Parkinson's because it does not reverse like that. My father knows that when he does not get his virgin coconut oil, the tremors return. What can I say?

Donna

My husband is 62 and has been showing signs the last couple of years of having Parkinson's disease. My husband has had hand tremors for some time now and his hands were also getting very stiff. He also showed some signs of confusion at times. He had spells where his whole body would hurt. And sometimes, when he was tired, he would kind of shuffle as he walked.

He started the program outlined in your book *Stop Alzheimer's Now* and I just have to share with you the results so far. We have stayed on the plan now for five weeks. This past week all of his hand tremors have stopped! His stiffness in his hands is gone! He has lost 20 pounds! All his body aches are gone! He is happier and has more energy! He seems more alert. I want to thank you for the book and all of your research!

Susan G.

Alzheimer's usually surfaces sometime after the age of 60. The disease affects 1 in 8 people over the age of 65 and affects nearly half of those over 85. In a small number of people it occurs in their 40s or 50s.

Currently there is no effective medical treatment for the disease. Treatment focuses on reducing the severity of the symptoms, combined with providing services and support to make living with the disease more manageable.

Drugs currently used to treat Alzheimer's at best might slightly ease some of the symptoms but this is debatable, since the results are so subtle it isn't clearly evident. Even if the benefit were tiny, it might be better than nothing at all, except the side effects can be devastating. Dozens of side effects have been reported including nausea, diarrhea, insomnia, headaches, hallucinations, generalized pain, and even death.

One of the characteristics of Alzheimer's is chronic inflammation in the brain. Chronic inflammation disrupts normal glucose metabolism. Our cells use glucose as fuel to power metabolic functions. The hormone insulin is needed to shuttle glucose into the cells. However, inflammation interferes with this process causing insulin resistance. Insulin resistance is the hallmark feature of type 2 diabetes. Alzheimer's disease has been described as a form of diabetes—brain diabetes. As a consequence, the brain is unable to absorb the glucose it needs in order to function normally. Brain cells literally begin to starve to death. As a result, the brain rapidly ages and degenerates, leading to dementia.

Coconut oil provides an alternative treatment for Alzheimer's and other brain related conditions that offers hope without all of the adverse side effects. What is it that makes coconut oil so beneficial to brain health? It is the MCFAs. The two primary sources of fuel that power our cells are glucose and fatty acids. We get glucose primarily from eating carbohydrate-rich foods and fatty acids from eating fats and from the fats stored in our bodies. While most of the cells in our body can use either glucose or fatty acids, our brains rely heavily on glucose. Fatty acids are unable to pass through the blood-brain barrier to enter the brain and, therefore, cannot be used as fuel for the brain. In Alzheimer's, the brain cells are unable to effectively use glucose and so the brain degenerates.

Here is where coconut oil comes to the rescue. The MCFAs provide an alternative source of energy for the brain. The ordinary fats and found in our diet and that are stored in our fat cells are composed of LCFAs. These fatty acids are too large to pass through the blood-brain barrier. However, MCFAs, which are smaller than LCFAs, are able to pass though without problem, providing the brain with another source of fuel. In addition, the liver converts some of the MCFAs into another type of fuel called ketones, which are also able to pass through the blood-brain barrier. Although the Alzheimer's brain cannot absorb glucose efficiently, it can absorb MCFAs and ketones without problem. Coconut oil, therefore, provides the brain with a source of energy that can keep the brain cells alive and functioning, and even stimulate healing and repair that can calm inflammation and reverse insulin resistance.

The addition of coconut oil into the diet can produce very positive effects on the brain. In one study, for instance, Alzheimer's patients consumed a beverage containing MCFAs or a beverage made using an ordinary vegetable oil. Ninety minutes after drinking the beverage the patients were given a cognitive test. The patients who drank the beverage containing the MCFAs scored significantly better on the test than the other group.[97] This study was remarkable for three reasons. First, it demonstrated that consuming MCFAs had a significant positive effect on Alzheimer's patients. Second, the effect was almost immediate, within 90 minutes there was a measurable different in cognitive ability between the two groups. Third, it only took one dose of MCFAs to see significant improvement. No Alzheimer's drug or treatment has ever come close to achieving results like this.

In another study, coconut oil was shown to prevent the formation of the plaque deposits in brain tissue that are characteristic in Alzheimer's patients, thus protecting the brain from damage.[98]

Most all brain disorders involve chronic inflammation and insulin resistance to some extent including Parkinson's disease, ALS, stroke, traumatic brain injury, and others. All of these conditions can benefit from the use of coconut oil. For more information on using coconut oil and a brain regenerating diet to treat common brain disorders and improve memory see my book *Stop Alzheimer's Now!: How to Prevent and Reverse Dementia, Parkinson's, ALS, Multiple Sclerosis, and Other Neurodegenerative Disorders.*

Chapter 4

COCONUT OIL ON TRIAL

In recent years coconut oil has experienced a resurgence in interest. Many doctors and laypeople are now saying that coconut oil is one of the "good" fats and does not contribute to heart disease. For the past three decades coconut oil has been unjustly criticized as an artery clogging saturated fat. Many people, including much of the media, still blindly criticize it. Consequently, people are confused. Is it good or is it bad? What's the truth? It's about time we clear up this confusion and set the record straight.

If you were accused of committing a crime you would expect to receive a fair trial. Evidence would be presented by both the prosecution and the defense. After hearing the evidence, an impartial jury would decide whether you are guilty or not guilty. That is the fair way to determine the truth of the matter. If you were denied a defense attorney and only the prosecution was allowed to present their case, the trial would be one-sided and you would be found guilty and punished. You would be labeled a criminal for the rest of your life. Such a trial would be unfair and the *truth* would never be known. Coconut oil has been the victim of such a judgment. It has been accused of a crime by causing heart attacks in innocent victims. Up until now coconut oil has not had a fair trial. Only the prosecution has spoken. It is now time for the defense to speak up.

Let's briefly review the "evidence" used to support the contention that coconut oil contributes to heart disease. We can look at this as a court of law with coconut oil on trial accused of causing heart disease. To prove the accusation against coconut oil, the facts must be irrefutable or so overwhelming that it must convince a jury beyond reasonable doubt. Remember, the accused is always *innocent* until *proven* guilty. In this case, you are the jury. Let's see how the evidence against coconut oil stacks up.

In this "trial" the prosecution will present their evidence first, followed by a rebuttal from the defense. To avoid bias, unsubstantiated claims, or comments from unknowledgeable people, the only evidence accepted in this trial will be published studies, historical data, and testimonies from reliable witnesses. After all the evidence has been presented each side will make a brief summary statement. The verdict will follow.

SATURATED FATS AND CHOLESTEROL
Prosecution
Coconut oil is composed predominately of saturated fatty acids. In fact, 92 percent of the fatty acids in coconut oil are saturated, making it the most highly saturated of all the dietary fats. Saturated fat has been shown to raise cholesterol. Cholesterol is a recognized risk factor for heart disease. Therefore, coconut oil increases risk of heart disease.

Defense
It is true that some saturated fats raise blood cholesterol, but natural coconut oil when used in a normal diet does not have a negative effect on cholesterol. This finding has been consistently reported in several studies over the past four decades. As far back as 1959, Hashim and colleagues showed that adding coconut oil up to 21 percent of daily calories into the diets of hypercholesterolemic men (those with high cholesterol) did *not* raise their total cholesterol levels.[1] In fact, the subjects' blood cholesterol actually *fell* by an average of 29 percent. This is certainly not a cholesterol-raising effect.

The fact that 21 percent of the subjects' total calorie intake was from coconut oil is significant. The American Heart Association says we should limit total fat intake to 30 percent of calories and no more than 7 percent should be from saturated fat. Yet these subjects received 21 percent from highly saturated coconut oil, and still their blood cholesterol levels dropped.

Bierenbaum and colleagues had similar results. They followed 100 men for five years who had a documented history of heart disease. During this time their fat consumption was restricted to 28 percent of total calories. The subjects were divided into two treatment groups and a control group. Half of the fat consumed (14 percent) in the treatment groups consisted of one of two mixtures. One group received a 50/50 mixture of corn and safflower oils. The other group received a 50/50 mixture of coconut and peanut oils. At the end of five years both groups had *lower* total cholesterol than when they started and lower than the untreated control group.[2]

Prior and colleagues measured the cholesterol levels of the entire populations of two Polynesian islands. He chose these islands because of their high coconut consumption. Up to 50 percent of their daily calories came from coconut oil. Even with this extraordinarily high amount of coconut oil in their diet they did not have elevated cholesterol levels.[3]

A review of the medical literature reveals many studies indicating that natural coconut oil, when consumed as part of the diet as it normally would be, does not have an adverse effect on cholesterol levels.[4-7]

CHOLESTEROL IN ANIMAL STUDIES
Prosecution

There are studies that do show that coconut oil raises blood cholesterol levels. The medical literature reports many studies on the cholesterol-raising effects of coconut oil on rabbits, chickens, and other animals.[8]

In fact, coconut oil is used by researchers to induce hypercholesterolemia (high cholesterol) in animals used in medical research.

Defense

Coconut oil is often criticized as being hypercholesterolemic based on animal studies. Indeed, many animal studies do show a cholesterol-raising effect with coconut oil feeding. However, several problems are associated with these studies.

In most of these studies the animals are not given a natural diet but are fed lab formulas. These formulas contain mixtures of fats, proteins, starch, sugar, fiber, and other components in order to manipulate and control the diet. Some of these components such as fat and sugar can comprise an enormous amount of the diet, far more than what the animals would ever get in nature. When you start feeding animals man-made diets anything can happen and what does happen isn't a reliable reflection on what goes on in the real world.

Another problem is that you cannot always use animal studies as examples of human physiology. What happens in the laboratory with animals eating experimental foods cannot always be extrapolated to humans eating a natural diet. Animals process, digest, and metabolize foods differently than humans. When rabbits, which are vegetarians, are fed meat products, cholesterol, or saturated fat, you cannot expect their response to be the same as humans, which are omnivores and have the physiology capable of digesting cholesterol and saturated fats. For instance, in humans, fish oils rich in omega-3 fatty acids are believed to provide protection against heart disease. In hamsters, however, they raise cholesterol in comparison to coconut oil.[9] If you extrapolated this result to humans, it would mean that fish oils, compared to coconut oil, promote heart disease because they are hypercholesterolemic. If you want to induce high cholesterol in a hamster, feed it fish oil, but does that mean fish oil causes high cholesterol or heart disease in humans? Not necessarily. So you can't say coconut oil causes high cholesterol in humans because it might do so in a rabbit or a chicken.

Another common problem with many animal studies is that the coconut oil used is not natural. It is *hydrogenated* coconut oil. Any result you get using hydrogenated coconut oil does not reflect the response you would get using natural, non-adulterated coconut oil.

CHOLESTEROL IN HUMAN STUDIES
Prosecution
There are many studies on human subjects that also demonstrate the hypercholesterolemic effect of coconut oil. Ahrens and colleagues performed one of the first studies documenting the effects of coconut oil on blood cholesterol in 1957.[10] They fed controlled diets to native Bantus in South Africa. Subjects were given 100 grams (½ cup) of one of several fats in a mixed diet. They found that coconut oil raised cholesterol levels whereas corn oil lowered them. It was this experiment that first sounded the alarm against coconut oil. Many studies since then have supported Ahrens' findings.

Defense
Ahrens' study had a serious flaw, which was repeated in other studies supporting the idea that coconut oil raised total cholesterol in humans. The problem is that Ahrens did not use natural coconut oil. He used *hydrogenated* coconut oil. Each one of his subjects consumed a half-cup of hydrogenated coconut oil every day. No wonder their cholesterol levels rose. *All* hydrogenated vegetables oils raise cholesterol, including hydrogenated soybean and corn oils. So these studies do *not* prove that coconut oil, natural coconut oil that is non-hydrogenated, contributes to heart disease.

Hydrogenation is a process in which unsaturated fatty acids are transformed into more saturated fatty acids. Through hydrogenation unsaturated fatty acids in vegetable oil can become saturated. The problem with this process is that when vegetable oils (including coconut oil) are hydrogenated, many of the fatty acids are transformed into *trans fatty acids*. These man-made fatty acids are foreign to the body and cause all manner of health problems. All hydrogenated vegetable oils contain trans fatty acids. A mountain of research now shows that hydrogenated oils from any source increases risk of heart disease.[11, 12]

Studies suggest that the risk of cardiovascular disease is increased more by the consumption of hydrogenated oils than by the consumption of any other type of fat.[13] DeRoos and colleagues showed that consumption of palm kernel oil, which is very similar to coconut oil, reduces risk of heart disease compared to hydrogenated soybean oil.[14] He even recommends the use of tropical oils as a safer alternative to hydrogenated oils.

ATHEROSCLEROSIS AND EFA DEFICIENCY
Prosecution
Ahrens and others found that coconut oil feeding in both human and animal studies not only raises cholesterol but also causes atherosclerosis. These studies provide evidence that coconut is both hypercholesterolemic and atherogenic (cause hardening of the arteries) and, therefore, contributes to the development of heart disease.

Defense
Again you cannot rely on these studies because they all used hydrogenated coconut oil, not natural coconut oil. Another very serious problem with many of the early studies with coconut oil is that researchers often fed test animals diets completely devoid of essential fatty acids (EFA). As a consequence, the animals became severely diseased due to an EFA deficiency. This diseased condition was misinterpreted as being caused by coconut oil.

Researchers fed test animals diets in which the sole source of fat was from hydrogenated coconut oil. Coconut oil has a small amount of EFA, only 2.5 percent. When coconut oil is hydrogenated these essential fatty acids are destroyed, leaving the oil completely void of all essential fatty acids. When test animals are given diets over a period of time that are missing all essential fatty acids, they consequentially become sick. Symptoms associated with essential fatty acids deficiency include high cholesterol and atherosclerosis (hardening of the arteries). Essential fatty acid deficiency disease can be caused by *any* hydrogenated oil, including polyunsaturated vegetable oils, when given as the sole source of fat in the diet.[15] Essential fatty acid deficiency is even more damaging to the arteries than the trans fatty acids found in hydrogenated oils.

The damage caused by EFA deficiency has nothing to do with coconut oil. This fact was clearly demonstrated by Morin and colleagues. He tested two groups of rats. One group was given a fat-free diet deficient in essential fatty acids. The other group was given a diet containing an adequate amount of essential fatty acids. After 16 weeks both groups were put on a single diet that contained hydrogenated coconut oil as the sole source of fat. All of the animals that were initially given the essential fatty acid deficient diet at the beginning of the study developed atherosclerosis in the coronary artery. However, none of the rats that were given the essential fatty acids at the beginning of the study developed atherosclerosis, even after consuming hydrogenated coconut oil.[16] If coconut oil caused atherosclerosis both groups would have developed this problem.

In another study dogs were fed 16 percent of their diet by weight as hydrogenated coconut oil supplemented with 5 percent cholesterol. The dogs all developed severe atherosclerosis. A second group of dogs were fed an identical diet except that 4 percent of the hydrogenated coconut oil was replaced by safflower oil, which supplied a small amount of essential fatty acids. The researchers reported that the second group of dogs were completely protected from the atherogenic process. Obviously, coconut oil did not cause the atherosclerosis in the first group of dogs. Essential fatty acid deficiency was credited as the cause of the atherogenicity.[17]

As researchers gradually became aware of essential fatty acid deficiencies in their research they attempted to correct for this problem. However, instead of using natural coconut oil, which contains a small amount of essential fatty acids they continued to use hydrogenated coconut oil but added a small amount of polyunsaturated oil to the test diets. The differences between cis (normal) fatty acids and trans (transformed) fatty acids were not generally recognized for many years. Researchers now use hydrogenated coconut oil to purposely induce EFA deficiency in test animals.[18]

After years of using hydrogenated coconut oil in cholesterol research, non-hydrogenated, natural coconut oil gained an undeserved bad reputation. These flawed studies are often quoted as "proof" that coconut oil causes heart disease or at least contributes to it. Even now, hydrogenated coconut oil is still being used in many studies, which continues to cloud the issue and cause confusion. Most researchers do it purposely to induce a cholesterol-raising effect when evaluating other dietary parameters. They don't have to use hydrogenated coconut oil. They can use hydrogenated soybean oil or hydrogenated safflower oil and depending on the degree of hydrogenation can get the same cholesterol-raising and atherogenic effects. Hydrogenated coconut oil is generally preferred because the smaller MCTs tend to mix better with test diets.

Often, studies don't identify if researchers used hydrogenated or natural coconut oil. This oversight was more of a problem in the past when researchers didn't know that the difference mattered. In older studies if a distinction wasn't made, then hydrogenated oil was probably used. Even when authors do indicate whether they use hydrogenated or non-hydrogenated coconut oil in a study, if you read only an abstract you might not know which was used because it often isn't stated. Abstracts are brief summaries of published studies and don't always reveal these details. You would have to read the entire article to find out.

FRACTIONATED COCONUT OIL
Prosecution

Even studies that don't use hydrogenated oils suggest that coconut oil is hypercholesterolemic. When the individual saturated fatty acids in coconut oil are evaluated, they often show a cholesterol-raising effect. Therefore coconut oil, which is composed mostly of saturated fatty acids, raises cholesterol. For example, researchers from the University of Texas Southwestern have shown that when MCT oil was fed to human volunteers it raised LDL (bad) cholesterol.[19] MCT oil is composed entirely of capric and caprylic acids, two saturated medium-chain fatty acids from coconut oil. The researchers concluded that contrary to previous studies that indicate that medium-chain triglycerides do not negatively affect cholesterol, their study indicated that they do.

Defense

You can't say coconut oil has a cholesterol-raising effect based on the evaluation of only one or two fatty acids. Like hydrogenated oil, MCT oil is *not* the same as natural coconut oil. MCT oil is fractionated coconut oil. It is a man-made oil containing only two fatty acids (i.e., caprylic and capric). Natural coconut oil contains at least 10 different fatty acids. The majority of these fatty acids are medium-chain, but it also includes short- and long-chain fatty acids, as well as oleic acid (a monounsaturated fatty acid) and linoleic acid (an essential polyunsaturated fatty acid). When MCT oil is used as the *only* dietary fat in a test diet, it too can produce effects that may be undesirable, just as hydrogenated coconut oil can.

The study cited above, like many others, is flawed. This study consisted of nine middle-aged men with mildly elevated cholesterol. They were each put on a *low-fat* diet, which was carefully prepared and controlled in a metabolic ward of the Dallas Veterans Affairs Medical Center. The subjects were tested for three weeks. MCT oil was the only fat added to the low-fat diet. The food itself contained very little fat, so the MCT oil supplied essentially all the fat the subjects ate. MCT, like hydrogenated oil, is completely devoid of all essential fatty acids. Therefore, the results weren't surprising when LDL cholesterol increased, because the diet was essential fatty acid deficient and caused symptoms of essential fatty acid deficiency.

The results of this study are contrary to those of many other studies, which have been designed to avoid the EFA deficiency problem. When adequate essential polyunsaturated fatty acids are included with a high MCT diet, heart disease risk actually decreases. Calabrese and others have shown that when MCT oil is added to a normal diet that supplies adequate essential fatty acids, it has a *favorable* effect on blood lipids and reduces overall cardiovascular risk.[20]

Even large amounts of MCT oil in the diet are not harmful when adequate EFAs are included. In fact, they are beneficial. Bourque and colleagues demonstrated that a diet containing as much as 50 percent of the fat from medium-chain triglycerides *lowers* cardiovascular risk.[21]

HYPERCHOLESTEROLEMIA IS RELATIVE
Prosecution

When you compare coconut oil with all other vegetable oils, it has the most detrimental effect on blood cholesterol. Even natural coconut oil is hypercholesterolemic compared to other oils.

Defense

Many cholesterol studies have compared *natural* coconut oil to other vegetable oils. The way the authors of these studies word their results often causes misunderstanding and confusion. Dietary oils are often labeled as either "hypercholesterolemic" meaning cholesterol-raising or "hypocholesterolemic" which signifies cholesterol lowering.

Coconut oil is often termed as being *hyper*cholesterolemic in *comparison* to polyunsaturated oils. The key word here is "comparison." Studies that supposedly show coconut oil having a hypercholesterolemic effect actually show that the oil was not as effective at lowering the serum cholesterol as was the polyunsaturated vegetable oils to which it was compared.

For example, if you looked at a person who stands 6 feet from head to toe, you would say that person is tall because he is well above average height. However, in comparison to most professional basketball players, many of which are nearly 7 feet tall, a 6-foot person would be considered short. If he was on a professional basketball team, he might even be nicknamed "Shorty." The fact that he is shorter than a few others doesn't make him short. He is still taller than average.

Let's look at olive oil. Olive oil has a cholesterol lowering effect. Safflower oil has a greater cholesterol lowering effect than olive oil. You can say that in comparison to safflower oil, olive oil has a cholesterol raising effect. This statement would make it appear that olive oil actually raises blood cholesterol, when in reality it doesn't.

The same situation exists with coconut oil in relation to other vegetable oils as far as total cholesterol is concerned. Coconut oil is referred to as being *hyper*cholesterolemic (cholesterol-raising) only in comparison to polyunsaturated oils. However, when compared to other saturated fats and hydrogenated vegetable oils, which raise serum cholesterol, coconut oil is *hypo*cholesterolemic (cholesterol lowering). In truth, coconut oil is neither. It generally has little effect on total cholesterol in humans.

RISK FACTORS FOR HEART DISEASE
Prosecution
Certain studies on humans suggest that natural coconut oil increases total blood cholesterol. For example, Ng and colleagues fed coconut oil to a group of volunteers and total cholesterol increased by as much as 17 percent.[22] Tholstrup and colleagues reported an increase of 16.2 mg/dl when palm kernel oil, which is very similar to coconut oil, was added to volunteers' diets.[23] According to these studies coconut oil consumption increases total cholesterol, and therefore, it also increases the risk for heart disease.

Defense
Coconut oil may have slightly varying effects on total cholesterol. The studies cited by the Prosecution show it appears to increase blood cholesterol. Other studies, some of which were cited earlier, have shown a decrease. In general the effects on total cholesterol are neutral.

The studies that show an apparent negative effect on cholesterol are misleading. When you evaluate *all* the data in the above studies you find that coconut oil and palm kernel oil have a positive overall effect on cholesterol. While total cholesterol may increase, this increase is due primarily to an increase in HDL cholesterol—the good cholesterol that *reduces* risk of heart disease.

Measurements of total cholesterol include both HDL (good) cholesterol and LDL (bad) cholesterol. If you don't know how much of the total cholesterol is HDL and how much is LDL you really don't know what your heart disease risk is. A far more accurate measure of heart disease risk is the cholesterol ratio (total cholesterol/HDL). You can have high total cholesterol but a low risk for heart disease if you also have a low cholesterol ratio. So a person who has a total cholesterol reading of say 240 (which is considered high) may have a lower risk than a person with a total cholesterol of 200 (which is considered normal) because the first person has more HDL (good) cholesterol and a lower cholesterol ratio.

The studies the Prosecution cited by Ng and Tholstrup show that although coconut oil increased total cholesterol in volunteers, it also increased HDL and lowered the cholesterol ratio thus *reducing* the risk of heart disease!

In Ng's study the cholesterol ratio was reduced from 2.51 to 2.42. In the Tholstrup study the ratio was reduced from 3.08 to 2.69. Both studies show a favorable change. The cholesterol ratio is considered to be a far more accurate indicator of heart disease risk than total cholesterol; therefore, coconut oil does not have a negative effect on cholesterol levels.

Actually, cholesterol levels are meaningless here. They don't prove anything. Even if coconut did raise blood cholesterol that wouldn't prove that coconut oil caused heart disease. Why? Because, contrary to popular belief, high blood cholesterol does not *cause* heart disease. If high cholesterol caused heart disease everyone with high cholesterol would have heart disease and die of heart attacks or strokes. But they don't. Many people with cholesterol levels well above 240 have no symptoms or signs of heart disease and lead full active, healthy lives. On the other hand, at least half of all those who suffer a heart attack have normal or below normal cholesterol levels.

Doctors don't know exactly what causes heart disease. If they did, then they could do something to stop it. But heart disease is our number one killer and still going strong. We haven't stopped it despite cholesterol education, low-fat dieting, cholesterol-lowering drugs, and all the wonders of medical science.

The belief that cholesterol causes heart disease is a common misconception perpetuated to a great deal by the food and drug industries to encourage sales of low-fat foods and cholesterol-lowering drugs.

In truth, cholesterol is only a marker or "risk factor" for heart disease. Other risk factors for heart disease include smoking, age, blood pressure, lack of exercise, and diabetes. Even gender is a risk factor for heart disease since males have higher disease rates, but that doesn't mean that being a male *causes* heart disease. None of these risk factors necessarily cause heart disease. Their presence only indicates an increased risk or chance for the disease. Many people believe that cholesterol has little or no affect on heart disease and is merely an innocent bystander. It's like going to the scene of a crime. Simply because police officers are present doesn't mean they caused the crime. So a measurement of total blood cholesterol level cannot be considered proof.

The real issue here is not how coconut affects cholesterol, but whether it causes heart disease. Remember that coconut oil is not on trial for its effect on cholesterol, it's on trial for causing heart disease. Even if it did raise cholesterol, that doesn't mean it's guilty of causing heart disease.

All the evidence given so far against coconut oil has been based on cholesterol levels. This approach has proven to be fruitless as there is insufficient evidence to show a negative effect on cholesterol. Just about the only way you could prove that coconut oil caused heart disease is to see if people who consume the oil suffer more from clogged arteries and heart attacks. I would like to see the Prosecution provide some real evidence to show that coconut oil causes heart disease.

HEART DISEASE DEATH RATES
Prosecution
Studies indicate that people who eat the most saturated fat have the highest heart disease death rates. Ancel Keys showed in his Seven Country study that the more fat people ate, the higher their death rate from heart disease.[24]

Defense

You cannot equate coconut oil to other fats, not even saturated fats because they are not the same. Population studies show that those people who eat coconut oil as a part of their daily diets have a low incidence of heart disease. In fact, those people who eat the most coconut oil have the lowest heart disease rates in the world. In the Philippines, for example, coconut and coconut oil are staples in the diet for many people. The heart disease death rate in the Philippines is one of the lowest, even lower than Japan, which has the highest life expectancy of any First World country. The Bicol region of the Philippines has the highest coconut oil consumption in the country, yet has the lowest heart disease rate.[25] In Sri Lanka where coconut oil has traditionally been the predominant dietary fat, the death rate due to heart disease has been only 1 out of every 100,000.[26] The same pattern is seen in Thailand, Indonesia, Fiji, and other coconut eating communities in the world. Population studies clearly show that coconut oil consumption does not contribute to heart disease.

According to the Prosecution, if coconut oil causes heart disease, every population that is a heavy coconut consumer should have a high death rate from heart disease. I would challenge the Prosecution to identify any such population.

Prosecution

Heart disease has been rising all around the world even in coconut growing regions.

Defense

The reason for this is that coconut oil consumption worldwide has been declining due to the mistaken belief that it contributes to heart disease. Processed vegetable oil and hydrogenated oil consumption has been increasing. Even though heart disease rates in places like the Philippines has been increasing, the effects are seen more in urban dwellers who eat a high amount of imported foods, including processed vegetable oils. On a whole, the death rate for heart disease in the Philippines is still far lower than that in the United States and most of Europe. As long as these people eat coconut oil as their main source of fat, their heart disease rates remain relatively low.

TESTIMONY OF EXPERT WITNESSES
Judge

Is there any more evidence the Prosecution would like to present?

Prosecution

We have numerous medical professionals, physicians and scientists, who can testify that coconut oil contributes to heart disease. These professionals routinely recommend the consumption of polyunsaturated vegetable oils as part of a heart healthy diet and the avoidance of saturated fats, particularly coconut oil. As health care professionals their opinions are highly respected.

Defense

The problem with the Prosecution's witnesses is that they are not experts in lipid biochemistry and have neither clinical nor laboratory experience working with natural coconut oil. Like most other people in the health care profession, their opinions are influenced by flawed studies that use hydrogenated coconut oil. Most doctors know little if anything about MCTs and their effect on human physiology. Most doctors don't even know there is more than one type of saturated fat. Doctors receive very little training in diet and nutrition in medical school and, therefore, are not experts in this field. For these reasons, the vast majority of medical professionals are not qualified as expert witnesses regarding the health aspects of coconut oil.

Judge

Is there any more evidence the Defense would like to present?

Defense

Yes. We would like to call several expert witnesses, lipid researchers and doctors, who have first-hand experience working with natural coconut oil in human research. These men and women have studied the effects of coconut oil as part of a natural diet. We will let them each make a statement.

"Humans tend to eat mixtures of fats, yet very rarely have dietary lipids been examined as mixtures. Early animal experiments are of limited value because these animals developed essential fatty acid deficiency. This would have been avoided by feeding mixtures of fats, as the interaction of different fatty acids might not be simply additive. In the few trials of coconut oil as part of a mixed fat diet, a hypercholesterolemic response was not observed...Coconut oil has historically been misrepresented, and the scientific community, therefore, must be educated on its true metabolic process and effect on atherogenesis."
—George L. Blackburn, M.D., Ph.D.,
Edward A. Mascioli, M.D.,
Marilyn Kowalchuk, M.S., R.D.,
Vigen K. Babayan, Ph.D.,
Bruce R. Bistrian, M.D., Ph.D.
Research team at Harvard Medical School, Boston MA

"Population studies show that dietary coconut oil does not lead to high serum cholesterol nor to high coronary heart disease mortality or morbidity rate."
—Hans Kaunitz, M.D.
Clinical Professor of Pathology
Columbia University, College of Physicians & Surgeons

"Epidemiological data fail to show any cholesterogenic or atherogenic effects of high coconut oil intake in human populations. There is no evidence whatever that coconut consuming peoples suffer from heart disease as a result of coconut oil. In fact, it even appears that the coconut oil consumers have lower heart disease rates than non-coconut consumers. Certainly, coconut oil appears to enhance HDL (good cholesterol) levels to keep the LDL:HDL ratio desirably low."
—Conrado S. Dayrit, M.D., F.P.C.P., F.P.C.C., F.A.C.C.
Professor Emeritus, College of Medicine
University of the Philippines

"It is the long chain fatty acids present in animal food and milk products that contribute to production of cholesterol in the liver and in this respect coconut oil is considered a neutral oil. It neither increases the serum cholesterol level nor reduces the serum cholesterol level."
—D.P. Atukorale, M.D., F.R.C.P., F.A.C.C., F.C.C.P.

"Coconuts are used extensively in the diet in many different parts of the world. These populations are in the developing world where coronary heart disease is uncommon or rare."
—Ian A Prior, M.D., F.R.C.P., F.R.A.C.P.

"Incorporation of coconut oil in the diet will increase high density lipoprotein (HDL) levels in the blood. As you know HDL is the good cholesterol complex and should be high while the LDL should be low. Using coconut oil and coconut butter in your cooking would be a good idea."
—Laszlo I. Belenyessy, M.D.

Prosecution
Seeing that the Defense's witnesses are qualified and have extensive experience in lipid biochemistry and research involving coconut oil consumption, we have no further questions.

CLOSING STATEMENTS

Prosecution

Most medical professionals are of the opinion that saturated fats raise blood cholesterol and promote atherosclerosis and heart disease. Of all the dietary fats, coconut oil has the highest saturated fat content. Therefore, by its nature it should have a negative effect on cholesterol. Since cholesterol is a known risk factor for heart disease, coconut oil consumption promotes, if not causes, heart disease.

Defense

The Prosecution has just given the typical reasoning why most people mistakenly believe coconut oil causes heart disease.

Coconut oil does contain a high amount of saturated fat, but the saturated fat is predominately MCTs. Medium-chain triglycerides are processed and metabolized by the human body differently from other saturated fats and, therefore, do not have the same effect that other fats do. MCTs are converted into MCFAs and used by the body as a source of fuel to produce energy. They are not packaged into lipoproteins (e.g., VLDL and LDL cholesterol) to the degree or circulate in the bloodstream as much as other fats. Therefore, they do not raise blood cholesterol or cause atherosclerosis.

Studies in the past that have given coconut oil a bad name were flawed or misinterpreted. Animal studies are not reliable because fat metabolism in animals is often very different than that of humans. Both animal and human studies often used hydrogenated coconut oil and, therefore, are unreliable because trans fatty acids from any source raise cholesterol. Hydrogenated vegetable oils are recognized as a bigger threat than saturated fats in terms of promoting heart disease. Diets where hydrogenated or fractionated coconut oil is the sole source of fat leads to essential fatty acid deficiency, which is characterized by elevated cholesterol and the formation of atherosclerosis. When compared to other vegetable oils, coconut oil has been labeled hypercholesterolemic because it does not lower blood cholesterol as much as these other oils. That does not mean it has a true hypercholesterolemic effect, only a relative one in comparison to vegetable oils. Even if coconut oil did raise cholesterol this wouldn't prove that it caused heart disease. Studies suggest that coconut oil increases HDL (good) cholesterol while lowering the cholesterol ratio, thus reducing risk of heart disease.

Studies involving humans who use natural coconut oil as part of a normal diet show no adverse effects on blood cholesterol. Populations that consume significant amounts of coconut oil in their daily diets all have low rates of heart disease.

Finally, the testimonies of expert witnesses have sided with the Defense proclaiming coconut oil's innocence.

Is there sufficient evidence to show that coconut oil causes heart disease? Judging from the evidence presented, there isn't. Studies used as evidence for the Prosecution have all been flawed or misinterpreted. Furthermore, the Prosecution has failed to find a single population in the entire world that depends on coconut or coconut oil in their daily diet that has a high incidence of heart disease. When you consider all the facts, there is absolutely no real evidence that coconut oil consumption causes or in any way contributes to heart disease.

GUILTY OR NOT GUILTY
Judge

You have seen the evidence against coconut oil. As the jury you must decide if coconut oil is guilty of causing heart disease or not. Keep in mind that in a court of law the accused is always assumed to be innocent until proven guilty. Is there enough evidence against coconut oil to prove it guilty? You decide.

From the evidence provided above, it should be obvious that there is not enough credible evidence to convict coconut oil as being a deadly artery-clogging fat, as it has been so often called. As you will see in the following chapter, not only is coconut oil innocent of causing heart disease, but it actually protects against it. The food that has been condemned for so many years as causing heart disease actually helps prevent it.

Cholesterol

After 5 months of 3 tablespoons daily, my cholesterol stayed the same at 187, LDL 68, HDL 93, and VLDL 24.
Nancy

Two weeks ago I went and had a test done at the local clinic and my total cholesterol was 175, triglycerides were 71 and blood sugar 85. The nurse was floored with my answer when she asked what kind of oils we used. Her jaw really dropped when I mentioned coconut oil! She said I should change my eating habits. So I asked her how many 52-year-old guys does she come across that have numbers this good and are on no medications of any type.
Chuck

Chapter 5

COCONUT OIL IS GOOD FOR YOUR HEART

CARDIOVASCULAR DISEASE

Chances are you will die from some form of cardiovascular disease. Most people do. Sadly, most cardiovascular diseases are preventable. But once the disease has progressed to the point where you know you have it, it's usually too late. Little can be done through conventional treatments to save you. The best protection against cardiovascular disease is prevention. In most cases, it can be prevented.

Cardiovascular disease or heart disease, as it is commonly called, is a general term for all disorders of the heart and blood vessels. Atherosclerosis (hardening of the arteries) is by far the most common cardiovascular disease. It is of great concern because it sets the stage for hypertension (high blood pressure), heart attack, and stroke. Cardiovascular disease is and has been the leading cause of death in Western countries for decades.

Heart disease gives no warning, and most people who have the disease don't even know it. The first sign or symptom of heart disease is often a heart attack, a third of which are fatal. Heart attacks can come without any prior symptoms or warning. More people die of heart attacks than any other cause. It is the number one killer worldwide, killing 7.2 million people a year. In the United States someone dies of a heart attack every 40 seconds.

Although heart attacks can occur without warning, they don't just happen. The conditions that lead to a heart attack build up slowly over many years. Heart attacks, strokes, and other serious cardiovascular disorders, are usually a consequence of atherosclerosis. Atherosclerosis is a process in which hardened fatty material known as plaque is deposited inside the artery walls.

If you asked most people what causes atherosclerosis, they will probably tell you it was from having too much cholesterol in the blood. Cholesterol doesn't simply come dancing freely down the artery and suddenly decide to stick somewhere. In fact, cholesterol isn't even necessary for atherosclerosis or the formation of plaque. Contrary to popular belief, the principle component of arterial plaque is not cholesterol or fat but protein. Some atherosclerotic arteries contain little or no cholesterol.

Atherosclerosis initially develops as a result of injury to the inner lining of the artery wall. The injury can be the result of any number of factors such as high blood pressure, infection, free radicals, etc. Small proteins in the blood, known as platelets, cause clots to form when they encounter an injury to blood vessels. Clotting is necessary to stop bleeding and facilitate healing. Injured cells release protein growth factors that stimulate growth of the muscle cells within the artery walls to repair the damage. If the cause of the injury persists or becomes chronic, a complex mixture of scar tissue, platelets, calcium, cholesterol, and triglycerides are incorporated into the site in an effort to heal the injury. This material is called plaque. Fibrous tissue, which is primarily protein, not cholesterol, forms the principle material in plaque. Calcium deposits harden the plaque, making the arteries brittle, which is a characteristic of atherosclerosis. This is why atherosclerosis is referred to as "hardening of the arteries." As plaque builds, the passageway within the arteries narrows, and blood flow becomes restricted.

Contrary to popular belief, plaque isn't simply plastered along the inside of the artery canal. It grows inside and is incorporated into the tissues of the artery wall. Arterial walls contain a layer of strong circular muscles that prevent the plaque from expanding outward. As the plaque grows, it has only one way to expand and that is by protruding into the opening of an artery canal. The artery slowly narrows, choking off blood flow.

Arteries damaged by plaque encourage clot formation. A clot, once formed, may remain attached to plaque in the artery and gradually enlarge until it completely blocks the flow of blood. A clot can also break loose and be carried by the blood into smaller vessels where it can become lodged, blocking blood flow. Arteries that are already narrowed by plaque are easily clogged by clots. When blood flow in the coronary artery, which feeds the heart, is blocked, it causes a heart attack. When the blockage occurs in the carotid artery going to the brain, it causes a stroke. Clogging in other arteries can lead to kidney failure and gangrene.

WHY PACIFIC ISLANDERS DON'T GET HEART DISEASE

A century ago heart disease was almost unheard of. By 1950 it had become the leading cause of death in the United States as well as in many European countries. Like a plague it has spread to every corner on earth and is now the world's number one killer. Traditionally, the islands of the Pacific have been relatively immune to this menace. Where people still depend on their traditional coconut-based diet, heart disease continues to be a rarity.

Most medical professionals believe that heart disease is a consequence of diet and lifestyle. So, if you eat the right types of food, you can prevent a heart attack. In this respect, coconut, and particularly coconut oil, appears to be an effective weapon against heart disease.

Epidemiological (population) studies have shown that coconut-eating populations around the world have a remarkable immunity to heart disease. This immunity isn't genetic but diet related. Shorland and colleagues showed that Polynesian populations with high coconut consumption have lower blood cholesterol levels and lower incidence of atherosclerosis than Europeans and islanders who consume a Westernized diet.[1]

A major study was done on the populations of two remote Pacific Islands—Pukapuka and Tokelau.[2] The entire populations of the islands took part in the study. The foods the people ate were carefully analyzed and their health evaluated. These people were chosen because they have remained relatively isolated from Western influences and maintained their traditional coconut-based diet. Coconut was their primary source of food and was eaten in one form or another at every meal and as a snack between meals. The two populations derived 63 and 34 percent of their calories from coconut. The coconut oil they consumed in their diet amounted to over 100 grams a day, the equivalent to about half a cup. The researchers found that there was no evidence of coronary heart disease nor was there any evidence of diabetes, cancer, hypothyroidism or other health problems common in Western society.

Despite the high amount of saturated fat in the islanders' diet, their cholesterol levels were much lower than expected. Using the Key's equation, which calculates cholesterol levels as a function of dietary fat intake, cholesterol levels were predicted. The islander's actual cholesterol levels, however, were on average 76 mg/dl lower than the predicted values—a huge difference.

Coconut plays a central role in the diet of the people in the South Pacific island of Papua New Guinea. As with other island populations these people have been eating coconut for generations without a single reported case of a heart attack. If coconut oil contributes to heart disease, as many people have been led to believe, these people should be riddled with heart attacks and strokes, yet heart disease was completely unknown here until 1964 when the first case was reported.[3] As the country has become more Westernized, coconut consumption has declined and heart disease cases have increased. All of these cases have been confined to major urban areas where dietary habits have become Westernized.

A series of studies on relatively isolated populations in Papua New Guinea that have maintained their traditional coconut-based diets have found these people to be completely free from all signs of heart disease. For example, in one of the studies with 203 individuals, researchers reported the "nonexistence of stroke and ischemic heart disease" even in people as old as 86 years of age.[4]

On the island of Kitava in Papua New Guinea, coconut is a dietary staple. These people represent a typical Pacific island population. A total of 1816 subjects participated in the study, ranging in age up to 96 years. Researchers reported that "stroke and ischemic heart disease appear to be absent in this population."[5]

All the inhabitants including the oldest members of the population, who were approaching 100 years of age, had low blood pressure. Fasting total cholesterol and LDL cholesterol were 10 to 30 percent lower in Kitavan males as compared with the Swedish population who consumes a diet slightly lower in saturated fat, but higher is so-called "heart healthy" monounsaturated and polyunsaturated fats.[6]

From the studies cited above, heavy coconut consumption does not appear to have any harmful effect and, from all indicators, seems to protect the people from heart disease even into old age. Pacific Islanders aren't the only ones who are protected from the ravages of heart disease; all of the populations around the world that depend heavily on coconut as a part of their diet have a very low incidence of heart disease.

In Sri Lanka, coconut has been the primary source of dietary fat for thousands of years. In 1978 the per capita consumption of coconut was equivalent to 120 nuts per year. At that time the country had the lowest rate of heart disease in the world. Only one out of every 100,000 deaths was attributed to heart disease. In the United States, where very little coconut is eaten, the heart disease death rate at the same time was at least 280 times higher!

Over the years, coconut consumption in Sri Lanka has decreased while the incidence of heart attacks has increased; in 1952 per capita consumption of coconut was 132 nuts, in 1991 it dropped to 90. Generally heart disease has been confined to urban areas where consumption of coconut has declined the most. In rural areas it remains the primary source of dietary fat. Among the aboriginal population in Sri Lanka coconut is a major source of food and coronary heart disease is completely unknown.[7]

In the coconut growing regions of southern India where large quantities of coconuts and coconut oil have traditionally been consumed, an average 2.3 out of 1,000 people suffered from coronary heart disease in 1979. A campaign against the use of coconut oil on the grounds that it was an "unhealthy" saturated fat and caused heart disease decreased coconut oil consumption during the 1980s. Processed vegetable oils and margarine replaced it in household use. As a result, by 1993 the heart disease rate tripled!

Many studies have shown that the Japanese have one of the longest life expectancies in the world. Part of this is due to their low rates of cancer and heart disease. From data supplied by the American Heart Association (AHA) the

CARDIOVASCULAR DISEASE DEATHS[1]

Country	Deaths
Russian Federation	1802
Hungary	1330
Romania	1283
Bulgaria	1250
Poland	1136
Czech Republic	997
Argentina	993
Mexico	973
Columbia	957
China	931
Scotland	906
Denmark	874
Korea	840
Ireland	815
United States	814
Portugal	773
Belgium	758
Northern Ireland	743
Germany	732
Finland	729
Netherlands	703
England/Wales	702
Canada	701
New Zealand	683
Israel	683
France	679
Norway	656
Austria	653
Greece	646
Spain	640
Italy	610
Sweden	596
Australia	577
Switzerland	559
Japan	548
Philippines	120[2]

Ages 35-74 Rate per 100,000 Population.

1. Death rates for total cardiovascular disease, coronary heart disease, and stroke in selected countries (most recent year available as of 2004). Source: American Heart Association.

2. Source: Dayrit, C.S. 2003. Coconut oil: atherogenic or not? *Philip J Cardiology* 31(3):97-104.

cardiovascular mortality rate in 35 countries is listed from highest to lowest in the table above. Of all the countries listed, Japan has the lowest death rate from cardiovascular disease. None of the countries listed, however, are major coconut consumers. Even the Japanese don't eat much coconut, but in the Philippines they do. The Philippines was not included in the main list because the AHA did not have data available for that country. In a study by Conrado Dayrit, M.D., published in the *Philippine Journal of Cardiology*, the cardiovascular disease death rate for the Philippines is given as 120 per 100,000.[8] This rate is even lower than Japan's. In fact, the cardiovascular disease death rate is less than a fourth of Japan's. In the Philippines where coconut consumption is greatest, heart disease is also lowest. The Bicol region of the Philippines has the highest intake of fat from coconut because they cook most food in coconut milk; 62.5 percent of the fat in their diet is from coconut. The Bicolanos have the lowest incidence of heart disease in the country.

Studies show that in populations where Western food intake is negligible and coconut consumption is high, stroke and heart disease are absent or rare.[9] Over the years it has been seen that when island populations abandon their native diets rich in coconut and embrace modern foods and lifestyles, they develop the same types of diseases seen in the West and heart disease rates rise. The more Westernized the people become, the more their diseases mimic those commonly found in the West.

Ian Prior, M.D., a cardiologist and director of the epidemiology unit at the Wellington Hospital in New Zealand, says this pattern has been very clearly demonstrated with Pacific Islanders. "The more an Islander takes on the ways of the West, the more prone he is to succumb to our degenerative diseases." He states that the further the Pacific natives move away from the diet of their ancestors "the closer they come to gout, diabetes, atherosclerosis, obesity, and hypertension."[10]

Is coconut the secret that protects Pacific Islanders against heart disease or is there something else? You might argue that it is the traditional diet as a whole that is protective and not just the coconut. This is a reasonable argument. Enough evidence, however, strongly suggests that coconut is a major reason why Pacific Islanders don't get heart disease. Islanders who eat more coconut than others have a lower risk of heart disease. This was illustrated in a study that compared two Polynesian populations from the Cook Islands. The two islands in the study were Pukapuka and Rarotonga. Both populations came from the same ethnic background. Although Rarotongans were influenced more by Western culture, the two populations ate basically the same types of foods and lived in similar environments and conditions. The main difference in their diet was the amount of coconut eaten. The Pukapukans ate more coconut and consumed a higher amount of fat. Seventy-five percent of the fat in the Pukapukan diet was from coconut oil. The Rarotongans derived 25 percent of their fat from coconut oil. Even though the Pukapukans ate more coconut oil and more total fat, their blood cholesterol levels were considerably lower than the Rarotongans. Cholesterol values for Pukapukans averaged 175 mg/dl, which is considered to be in the low risk range.[11] The higher amount of coconut in the

Pukapukans diet apparently improved cholesterol readings, thus lowering their risk of heart disease. The evidence showing that coconut oil is one of the secrets that keeps Pacific Islanders free from heart disease is presented in further detail throughout the rest of this chapter.

HOW COCONUT OIL PROTECTS
AGAINST HEART DISEASE

Coconut has been called the king of foods. It is used as both a food to sustain life and as a medicine to restore health. Tradition has it that eating the fruit of the coconut tree is one of the secrets to good health and a long life. Current medical research is now revealing the health restoring properties of this king of foods.

Ironically, coconut oil, which was once criticized as contributing to heart disease is now revealing itself as a powerful weapon against it. What is it about coconut oil that keeps heart disease at bay? Let's take a look at how coconut oil affects cardiovascular health.

After decades of research the cause of heart disease is still unknown. Researchers, however, have identified several factors that are often associated with heart disease. These are called risk factors. The more risk factors you have, the higher your chances of dying from a heart attack or stroke. The 12 most commonly recognized risk factors are:

Age	Blood Cholesterol Levels
Gender (being male)	Obesity and Overweight
Smoking	Diabetes
Stress	Hypertension
Lack of Exercise	Homocysteine Levels
Heredity	Arterial Inflammation

The first six—age, gender, smoking, stress, lack of exercise, and heredity—are unrelated to diet. So whether someone eats coconut oil or not, it won't affect these. The second six—blood cholesterol levels, obesity, diabetes, hypertension, homocysteine levels, and even arterial inflammation—are diet related. So these are the factors that could be influenced by coconut oil consumption. Let's look at how coconut oil affects each one of these recognized risk factors for heart disease.

Blood Cholesterol Levels

In the last chapter the relationship between cholesterol and coconut oil was covered extensively. You learned that natural coconut oil has little effect on total cholesterol. When coconut oil is altered by hydrogenation or fractionation, total cholesterol can be adversely affected, but natural coconut oil does not produce the same results.

Total blood cholesterol is the number you normally receive as test results. Cholesterol is generally expressed in milligrams per deciliter of blood (mg/dl). Total cholesterol is not a very accurate measure of heart disease risk. Only about half of the people who die of heart disease have elevated cholesterol levels. Sometimes people with low cholesterol die of heart attacks. Research shows that "80 percent of individuals who developed coronary artery disease (CAD) have a total plasma cholesterol value within the same range as those who do not develop CAD."[12] Therefore, you can't rely on total cholesterol values for an accurate indicator of heart disease risk.

A much more accurate indicator of risk is the cholesterol ratio.[13] Total cholesterol contains both good and bad cholesterol. Low-density lipoprotein (LDL) is considered the "bad" cholesterol because it is the cholesterol that is being deposited in the tissues throughout the body. High-density lipoprotein (HDL) is considered the "good" cholesterol because it is the cholesterol being removed from the body. So the more HDL (good) cholesterol you have, the lower your risk of heart disease. The cholesterol ratio is obtained by dividing total cholesterol by HDL cholesterol. For example, if a person has a total cholesterol of 200 mg/dl and an HDL cholesterol level of 50 mg/dl, the ratio would be stated as 200/50 or 4. The goal is to keep the ratio below 5; the optimum ratio is 3.2 or less (see table below).

CHOLESTEROL RATIO	
Total-C/HDL-C (mg/dl)	**Risk**
3.2 or less	low risk (optimal)
3.3 – 4.9	less than average risk
5.0	average risk
5.1 or greater	high risk

The reason that total cholesterol is an unreliable indicator of heart disease risk is that it includes both the good (HDL) and the bad (LDL) cholesterol. You don't know how much of each contributes to the total. You may have high total cholesterol and yet be at low risk because you have a larger proportion of HDL. For example, a total cholesterol reading of 320 would be considered extremely high. Yet if your HDL was 80, your risk would actually be below normal because your cholesterol ratio (total-C/HDL-C) would be 4. If your total cholesterol was only 180, which by itself is considered low risk, but your HDL was 32, your ratio would be 5.6, which indicates high risk. Therefore, you cannot depend on total cholesterol for an accurate measure of heart disease risk. The ratio of total cholesterol to HDL cholesterol is a far more accurate indicator.

Total cholesterol levels can vary depending on several factors including diet, medications, and lifestyle. Even the results from testing laboratories differ from one another. I've seen people who were overjoyed because their cholesterol levels dropped when they added coconut oil into their diets. I've also had people express concern because their total cholesterol levels rose when they began using coconut oil. Why is cholesterol increased in one individual but decreased in another? I believe the key to this puzzle is that coconut oil has a balancing or normalizing effect. If total cholesterol is too high, coconut oil tends to lower it. If it is too low, it tends to raise it. What's too high and what's too low varies from person to person. For example, a cholesterol level of 220 may be high for one person but just right for another. This may explain why so many people who have high cholesterol are free from heart disease while those with normal cholesterol levels have heart attacks.

This effect can also be explained by the fact that coconut oil tends to raise the HDL (good) cholesterol in most individuals. Consequently, total cholesterol may increase. In this case the increase in total cholesterol can be a good thing because it lowers (improves) the cholesterol ratio, thus reducing risk of heart disease.

Studies that have isolated lauric acid from coconut oil and tested its effect on cholesterol have shown that it tends to raise total cholesterol. Since lauric acid comprises about 50 percent of the fatty acids in coconut oil, some people have suggested that coconut oil too must raise cholesterol and, therefore, increase risk of heart disease. However, when you evaluate the data from these studies, you find that the rise in total cholesterol is due primarily to an increase in HDL (good) cholesterol.[14-18] Consequently, the cholesterol ratio is improved, thus reducing risk of heart disease.

Natural coconut oil, not just the lauric acid, also tends to increase HDL and improve the cholesterol ratio. Studies have shown that it has a more favorable effect on HDL levels than either monounsaturated fats or polyunsaturated fats.[19]

An interesting study was done by Mendis and colleagues on Sri Lankan male volunteers.[20] Coconut oil is commonly used throughout Sri Lanka. Cholesterol levels were measured in subjects whose normal diet included coconut oil. Subjects were given corn oil to replace the coconut oil in their diets. Cholesterol levels were again measured.

When subjects switched from using coconut oil to corn oil their total serum cholesterol decreased an average of 18.7 percent from 179.6 to 146.0

mg/dl. LDL (bad) cholesterol decreased 23.8 percent from 131.6 to 100.3 mg/dl. Both of these changes are considered good and, if taken by themselves, would suggest that corn oil is superior to coconut oil as far as heart health is concerned. However, when you include the HDL (good) cholesterol numbers the picture changes. HDL cholesterol *decreased* 41.4 percent from 43.4 to 25.4 mg/dl, which is not good. The cholesterol ratio (total-C/HDL-C) increased from 4.14 to 5.75, which also is not good. A ratio less than 5.0 is considered to be less than average risk. A ratio greater than 5.0 is considered high risk. When volunteers ate coconut oil their risk was below average at 4.14 mg/dl. When they switched to corn oil they were propelled into the high-risk range at 5.75 mg/dl. The results of this study showed that coconut oil is far more effective than corn oil at reducing risk of heart disease. If you only looked at total cholesterol values, as we most often do, the conclusion would be completely reversed. When interpreting cholesterol values, you need HDL readings to get the whole picture.

Cholesterol Values in Sri Lankan Males		
Cholesterol	Coconut Oil	Corn Oil (mg/dl)
Total	179.6	146.0
LDL	131.6	100.3
HDL	43.4	25.4
Total/HDL	4.14	5.75

Polyunsaturated and monounsaturated vegetable oils have long been viewed as heart healthy because they tend to lower total cholesterol levels. Coconut oil does not lower total cholesterol like these other oils do and so has been viewed as less desirable. What we now know is that coconut oil has a greater beneficial effect on HDL, and consequently, the cholesterol ratio.

In clinical trials involving LDL and HDL and their effects on atherosclerosis and heart attacks, researchers found that even small increases in HDL cholesterol could reduce the frequency of heart attack. For every 1 mg/dl increase in HDL, there is a 2 to 4 percent reduction in the risk of coronary heart disease. In the above study, the coconut oil group had an average HDL value 18 mg/dl higher than in the corn oil group. So coconut oil *reduced* the risk of heart disease over corn oil—a cholesterol lowering polyunsaturated oil—by an incredible 36 to 72 percent!

Studies comparing coconut oil with safflower and soybean oils have given similar results.[21, 22] Even if coconut oil consumption raises total cholesterol, it has a positive effect on HDL, lowering the cholesterol ratio and, therefore, reducing risk of heart disease.

Cholesterol Values

When people add coconut oil into their diets their total cholesterol levels may rise or fall slightly, but in either case their HDL (good) cholesterol usually increases and their heart disease risk decreases. Here are a few examples.

Case One

This woman added 1 tablespoon of coconut oil a day to her diet for three months. Before using coconut oil her total cholesterol was 168 mg/dl, afterwards it increased to 187 mg/dl. Her LDL (bad) cholesterol dropped from 96 mg/dl to 87 mg/dl. Her HDL (good) cholesterol jumped from 60 mg/dl to 85 mg/dl. Her cholesterol ratio dropped from 2.8 to 2.2. Although her total cholesterol rose slightly it was still in the desirable range. Her cholesterol ratio was in the optimal range both before and after using coconut oil but was even better afterwards. Compare values with those listed in the table on page 106.

Cholesterol	Before	After (mg/dl)
Total	168	187
LDL	96	87
HDL	60	85
Total/HDL	2.8	2.2

Case Two

A woman began using coconut oil to help lower her cholesterol. She added a large amount, 4 to 8 tablespoons, of coconut oil daily into her diet for two months. At first she was disappointed when she received her cholesterol numbers. Her total cholesterol was 271 (high) and her LDL (bad) cholesterol was 168 (also high). Her triglyceride level, however, was very low at 80 mg/dl (which is optimal). Based on these numbers, her doctor pressured her to start taking cholesterol-lowering medication. However, her HDL (good) cholesterol was 94 and her cholesterol ratio was only 2.9, which is in the optimal range and, according to these numbers, at very low risk. She didn't need to worry about her total cholesterol, nor did she need to use cholesterol-lowering drugs.

Case Three

A woman had a family history of high cholesterol. Family members had total cholesterol readings in excess of 400 mg/dl. After adding coconut oil into her diet her total cholesterol rose from 336 to 376. Her HDL (good) cholesterol nearly doubled from 65 to 120. Her cholesterol ratio dropped from a high risk value of 5.2 to a low risk value of 3.1, which is in the optimal range. Although she had a very high total cholesterol reading, her true risk was very low. Her blood pressure was optimal at 110/60.

Cholesterol	Before	After (mg/dl)
Total	336	376
HDL	65	120
Total/HDL	5.2	3.1

Obesity and Overweight

The incidence of heart disease is significantly increased in persons who are overweight or obese. Obesity is defined as anyone who is 20 percent or more overweight. Nearly 70 percent of the diagnosed cases of heart disease are related to obesity. The risk of death rises with increasing weight. Even moderate weight excess (10 to 20 pounds for a person of average height) increases the risk of death, particularly among adults ages 30 to 64 years.

Body weight has a direct influence on several risk factors for heart disease. High blood pressure is twice as common in adults who are obese than in those who maintain a healthy weight. Obesity is associated with elevated blood fat levels and decreased HDL (good) cholesterol. A weight gain of only 11 to 18 pounds doubles a person's risk of developing type 2 diabetes. Insulin resistance and hyperinsulinemia (high insulin levels), which are conditions associated with diabetes, increase with weight. Over 80 percent of the people with diabetes are overweight or obese.

Not only is obesity associated with these other risk factors, but it is a risk factor in itself. Long-term studies indicate that obesity is an independent risk factor for heart disease. This relation appears to exist for both men and women with minimal increases in weight.

Recommendations to reduce the risk of both heart disease and obesity usually include limiting fat consumption. For many fats this is probably a good idea. A gram of fat supplies more than twice as many calories as an equal amount of carbohydrate or protein. You could eat twice as much protein and carbohydrate rich foods as you can fatty foods for the same number of calories. Since dieting limits food consumption, hunger is a common problem. Eating foods that provide more bulk is more satisfying and makes dieting a little easier. The reasoning is that if you remove most of the fat from your meals, you will be able to eat more low-calorie foods to fill you up. If you are not hungry, you will be less inclined to overeat or to snack between meals.

How does coconut oil fit into this picture? As you learned in Chapter 3, coconut oil is known as a low-calorie fat that can help overweight people lose excess pounds. Although coconut oil has slightly fewer calories than other fats, it still has more than carbohydrate and protein. What makes coconut oil useful as a weight loss aid is that it satisfies hunger better than both carbohydrates and proteins. When coconut oil is added to foods, hunger is satisfied sooner and delayed longer between meals. Consequently, people tend to eat less food throughout the day and consume fewer calories. Coconut oil also has a stimulating effect on metabolism, which increases the rate at which calories are burned. Because of this stimulating effect, simply adding coconut oil into a meal will reduce the effective number of calories in that meal. As long as you don't overeat, coconut oil can stimulate metabolism, satisfy hunger, and help you lose excess weight. When combined with a sensible diet, coconut oil can be an effective aid in weight loss. Because coconut oil consumption promotes weight loss, it also reduces risk of heart disease.

Diabetes

Diabetics are at high risk for heart disease because of poor circulation and a tendency to develop atherosclerosis. Every cell in our bodies needs a continual supply of either glucose or fatty acids to fuel metabolic functions and keep them alive. If the cells can't get enough glucose they weaken and die. As cells die, capillaries and blood vessels deteriorate and atherosclerosis develops. The hormone insulin is important because it opens the door on the cell membrane to allow glucose and fatty acids in the bloodstream to enter. Without insulin glucose can't enter the cells. With diabetes cells are unable to get the nourishment they need.

The two most common types of diabetes are type 1 and type 2. Type 1 occurs when the pancreas is unable to produce enough insulin to meet the body's needs. In type 2 diabetes the pancreas may be able to produce a normal amount of insulin, but the body's cells have become unresponsive to it. This is called insulin resistance.

In both types of diabetes cells are deprived of nourishment. The lack of nourishment causes cells to weaken and die; blood vessels tend to degenerate causing circulation problems. Artery walls that become damaged develop plaque, which clogs the arteries, leading to heart attack and stroke—the two leading causes of death in diabetics. Damage to capillaries that feed the nerves can result in neuropathy (nerve damage). Diabetic neuropathy often affects the legs and feet, causing pain and numbness and, if left untreated, ulcers and gangrene. A lack of circulation to the eyes may lead to diabetic-induced blindness, and in the kidneys it may cause kidney disease.

A low-fat diet is generally recommended for diabetes because fats are believed to increase the risk of obesity and heart disease, both of which are associated with diabetes. However, coconut oil may be one of the best foods for diabetics. Glucose as well as long-chain fatty acids require insulin to enter the cells. Medium-chain fatty acids in coconut oil do not need insulin. They can pass through the cell membrane and enter without it. Not only do MCFAs pass through the cell membrane with ease, but they also penetrate the mitochondria without assistance. Mitochondria are the energy producing organs of the cell. They take glucose or fatty acids and transform them into the energy the cells require to carry on their metabolic processes and keep them alive. Mitochondria have a double membrane, making it impossible for glucose and fatty acids to enter without the aid of special carriers called carnitine transferase. Medium-chain fatty acids can penetrate the double mitochondrial membrane without the assistance of this enzyme.[23] They are also oxidized faster to carbon dioxide with energy liberation.

Therefore, they can provide cells with nourishment whether insulin is present or not. When you eat coconut oil, you give your cells an energy boost. If the pancreas is not producing enough insulin or if the cells are insulin resistant, it doesn't matter, MCFAs can still feed the cells. This keeps capillaries and blood vessels alive and healthy and helps prevent atherosclerosis from developing. For this reason, coconut oil improves the circulation and cardiovascular health of diabetics.

After the publication of my book *The Coconut Oil Miracle,* I received a call from a man in California. He introduced himself as Bill S. and told me he was a diabetic. The reason he called was to thank me for introducing him to coconut oil. He had read my book and was encouraged to try it. He told me that due to a lack of circulation caused by his diabetes, he had lost most of the feeling in his feet (neuropathy). For months his feet felt like dead stumps. With excitement in his voice he stated, "When I began using coconut oil, my feet came alive!" His circulation improved to the point that his feet literally came back to life.

Since then I've heard many others report similar experiences. "I have been diagnosed with type 2 diabetes and my blood sugar has been around the 600 range," says Edward K. "I did have a minor scrape on my lower right leg that has been trying to heal for a couple of months. My wife called it an ugly wound. Six years ago my feet started to get numb, starting with the large toe and, over the years, the feet would become more and more numb. I began taking around 3 to 4 tablespoons per day of coconut oil. Within 10 days the injury on my leg healed up totally. I am so happy because now I feel the feeling coming back. The numbness is leaving. I have more feeling now." He further adds, "I would say within 5 weeks I lost 20 pounds. I am still going and want to drop even more. My skin feels marvelous, and looks the best it ever has. My scaly feet, I was so ashamed of before, they are looking much nicer."

Obviously, coconut oil improves circulation. It does not clog arteries but opens them up. To my knowledge coconut oil is the only thing that can cure diabetic neuropathy. And it's a harmless, natural product.

Not only are MCFAs in coconut oil able to feed the cells without the need of insulin, they also help improve insulin secretion, insulin sensitivity, and glucose tolerance.[24, 25] Lauric and capric acids, which make up the majority of the fatty acids in coconut oil, enhance the ability of the pancreas to secrete insulin. All of the MCFAs in coconut oil stimulate metabolism, thereby increasing the production of insulin and the absorption of glucose into cells. This is good news for the many diabetics who depend on daily insulin injections. Coconut oil can help reduce their dependency on insulin medication.

Coconut oil also helps to regulate blood sugar. Part of the reason for this is that it slows down the emptying of the stomach so that sugars are released into the blood stream at a slower rate. Another reason is that it helps to improve insulin secretion and insulin sensitivity. Many diabetics report that when they

Diabetes

Virgin coconut oil has a substantial effect on blood sugar levels. My wife and daughter, both have type 2 diabetes, they measure their blood sugar levels at least three times a day. When they eat the wrong foods and their blood sugar levels get to 80-100 points above normal, they don't take extra medication, they take 2-3 tablespoons of the coconut oil directly from the bottle. Within a half hour their blood sugar levels will come back to normal.

Ed

I was diagnosed as type 2 diabetic and immediately put on Amaryl RX. I have been looking for a way to reverse this condition since diagnosed. I have found a world of info out there on various supplements and diet. But not from my doctor who just said "Welcome to the club" and told me to take my meds…Bottom line is this. I have been able to slowly remove myself from the RX and now control my blood sugar by diet, supplements and with coconut oil! Cool, huh? I do still check my blood sugar levels once or twice daily and they are as good and usually BETTER than when I was on the Amaryl RX!

Sharon

I know many people with both type I and type II diabetes who have been helped by using virgin coconut oil. They started slowly and increased the amount used with meals slowly while monitoring their sugars. If they have trouble getting enough into their diets, they use it as a skin moisturizer. I personally had the wonderful experience of helping a friend who had a VERY SICK diabetic keeshond get off of insulin. We added virgin coconut oil and a couple of other non-chemical, non-toxic whole food supplements to her daily routine, and that near-dead sweet puppy is now the bundle of energy that dogs are supposed to be.

The diabetes was induced by vaccinations, and she had also developed skin allergies. She had very rough skin with many patches where the hair had fallen out. (A partially bald keeshond is quite pathetic/pitiful.) She rubbed the oil on her skin as well as adding a small amount to her food-with WONDERFUL results in both skin and lowered blood sugar levels. With our treatment, we lowered her insulin demand by 85% in 3-4 days, and off from it entirely in about 2 weeks. It really was a miracle.

Debby

add coconut oil to their diets their blood sugar levels are better even when they eat sugary foods. If blood sugar levels get too high, instead of taking extra medication, some people eat a couple tablespoons of coconut oil and their blood sugar levels drop back to normal within a half hour or so.

One of the major factors involved in the development of type 2 diabetes is insulin resistance. MCFAs can help to reverse this condition. They also help to keep blood glucose levels under control. When glucose is not allowed to enter the cells, because the cells are insulin resistant, the cells send signals that they are starving for food. In response to these signals, the pancreas, if it is able, pumps out more insulin. Insulin levels in the blood rise. Since glucose isn't being absorbed efficiently, blood glucose levels also rise. This elevation of insulin and glucose contributes to what is known as metabolic syndrome, as well as many additional health problems including an increase in heart disease risk. When MCFAs enter cells, the signal to the pancreas to produce more insulin is switched off and insulin levels stabilize. Complications and risks associated with diabetes and blood sugar problems are reduced.

When we eat foods that are converted into glucose, blood sugar levels rise. Some foods raise blood sugar more than others. The glycemic index is a system of measuring the effect specific foods have on blood sugar. Sweet and starchy foods like white bread and sugar have a high glycemic index and, therefore, quickly raise blood sugar. Even sweet fruits like bananas have a high glycemic index. Diabetics must carefully monitor and limit the amount of high glycemic foods they eat. Coconut oil has a favorable effect on blood sugar with a glycemic index of 0. When it is added to other foods it *lowers* the glycemic index of these foods. Even when added to starchy foods or sweets, the glycemic index of these foods is significantly lowered.[26] Adding coconut oil to meals is an effective way to lower the glycemic index of foods and help control blood sugar in diabetics.

Island populations that eat coconut regularly do not experience diabetes.[27] This is interesting because the foods these people eat are loaded with sweet fruits (such as bananas and pineapple) and starchy vegetables—foods diabetics normally must limit because of their effect on blood sugar. Coconut appears to help balance insulin and blood glucose levels and prevent insulin resistance. In one study, for example, 164 islanders from Kitava age 20 to 86 were compared with a randomly selected group of 472 Swedish controls age 25 to 74. Insulin levels in the islanders were significantly lower than the Swedes for all ages. The mean insulin concentration in Kitavans was only 50 percent of that in Swedish subjects. Insulin levels reflect the degree to which insulin resistance has developed. The researchers noted that the islanders diet (which relied heavily on coconut) and lifestyle were the primary reasons for their lower insulin levels.[28]

For these reasons, coconut oil is absolutely the best fat for a diabetic to eat and should be a part of any diabetic's daily diet. Since coconut oil is helpful in reducing conditions associated with diabetes, including circulation problems and atherosclerosis, it also reduces the risk of heart disease.

Hypertension

Hypertension is the medical term for high blood pressure. Blood is transported through the body by way of the arteries. Blood pressure is the force of the blood pushing against the walls of the arteries. Each time the heart beats (about 60 to 70 times a minute at rest), it pumps blood into the arteries.

High blood pressure is called "the silent killer" because it usually has no obvious symptoms. Some people may not know they have it until they have trouble with their heart, brain, or kidneys. High blood pressure puts a strain on the heart, causing it to grow larger, which may lead to heart failure. Excessive pressure against artery walls causes minute injuries that lead to chronic inflammation and the development of atherosclerosis. Atherosclerosis can lead to heart attack or stroke.

Chronic elevated blood pressure or hypertension is the most prevalent form of cardiovascular disease; in the United States it is believed to affect more than a third of the entire adult population. It contributes to half a million strokes and over a million heart attacks each year. The higher the blood pressure is above normal, the greater the risk of heart disease. High blood pressure is one of the strongest risk factors for heart disease.

Atherosclerosis is characterized by plaque that develops in the walls of the arteries. Plaque consists of a mixture of scar tissue, calcium, and fatty deposits. Plaque gradually builds, narrowing the passage through which the blood flows. Calcium deposits harden the artery and reduce its elasticity. Normally, the arteries expand with each heartbeat to accommodate the pulses of the blood that flow through them. Arteries that are hardened and narrowed by plaque cannot expand, so blood pressure rises. The increased pressure puts a strain on the heart and damages the artery walls further. Lesions develop in the artery wall. This is where plaques are especially likely to form, thus making the development of atherosclerosis a self-accelerating process.

Many things influence blood pressure. One of these is dietary fat, particularly polyunsaturated fats. Polyunsaturated fatty acids are classified into two main groups, namely omega-6 and omega-3. Both are converted into prostaglandins—hormone like substances that influence the way our bodies function. Omega-6 fatty acids are the fats found in most vegetable oils. Soybean, corn, safflower, and most other vegetable oils are composed predominately of omega-6 fatty acids. These fats are converted by the body into prostaglandins that constrict blood vessels, increase inflammatory response, and increase blood platelet stickiness, all of which increase blood pressure and promote atherosclerosis.

Omega-3 fatty acids, which are found in abundance in flaxseed and fish oils, are converted into prostaglandins that have just the opposite effect. These prostaglandins dilate blood vessels, reduce inflammatory response, and reduce blood platelet stickiness, all of which help lower blood pressure. This is why flaxseed and fish oils are regarded as heart healthy.

Medium-chain fatty acids in coconut oil are *not* transformed into prostaglandins. Therefore, they do not have the negative effects omega-6 fatty acids have or the positive effects of omega-3 fatty acids. This is good. Let me explain. By far the majority of the fats in our modern diet are composed of omega-6 fatty acids. If you eat any type of cooking oil, margarine, shortening, or any packaged or frozen food, you are consuming omega-6 fatty acids. The typical Western diet is loaded with omega-6 fatty acids. Since the prostaglandins produced by omega-6 fatty acids promote high blood pressure, it is no wonder that one third of the population has this problem.

The omega-3 fatty acids in flaxseed and fish oils can help balance or reverse the detrimental effects of omega-6 fatty acids. Omega-3 fatty acids, however, are very sensitive to oxidation and go rancid quickly. Heat, oxygen, and sunlight quickly oxidize these delicate fatty acids, creating toxic by-products that are worse than the effects of excess omega-6. This is why you never use them for cooking and must use them within a few weeks after purchase. Omega-3 fatty acids are usually taken as dietary supplements rather than eaten as food. Consequently, most people don't get enough omega-3 fatty acids to counterbalance the effects of the omega-6 fatty acids that are consumed in nearly every meal.

Coconut oil, being composed predominately of MCFAs, can dilute the effects of omega-6 fatty acids. When used in place of other oils in food preparation, the amount of omega-6 fatty acids in the diet is reduced considerably. Coconut oil is very resistant to oxidation and rancidity and, therefore, it makes an ideal cooking oil.

Using coconut oil for all your cooking and food preparation needs reduces the amount of omega-6 fatty acids in your diet, thus reducing the effects of prostaglandins that raise blood pressure. If blood pressure is elevated due to the over consumption of omega-6 fatty acids, simply removing these fats from the diet will lower it. This is exactly what people experience when they substitute coconut oil for the other oils they have been using in their diet.

This explains a conflicting observation reported by some coconut oil users. Many hypertensive people have reported a significant drop in blood pressure when they began using coconut oil. Others have reported little or no effect. The question they asked is why would it affect some people and not others? The answer is that if you eat a lot of packaged convenience foods or use ordinary cooking oil in your diet, coconut oil may have a significant effect at lowering your blood pressure. If you don't eat these types of foods, the effect will be less.

Polyunsaturated cooking oils aren't the only oils that negatively affect blood pressure. Monounsaturated fats such as canola and olive oils also raise blood pressure by increasing platelet stickiness.[29] Our blood contains special proteins called platelets. When these platelets come into contact with injuries along the artery wall they become sticky, causing blood cells to cling together and form clots. This is good if we have a wound because it prevents excessive bleeding and aids in healing. However, if the blood is continually sticky, it becomes "thick," making it harder to circulate through the narrow passageways of the arteries and veins. Blood pressure increases.

Coconut oil does not directly affect platelet stickiness either one way or the other. Even when hydrogenated, coconut oil demonstrates less of an effect than corn oil.[30] Fish oil reduces platelet stickiness whereas polyunsaturated vegetable oils, like corn oil, increase it. Coconut oil is in between.[31]

Coconut oil, however, may have more than just a benign effect on blood pressure. Another factor that affects blood pressure is insulin resistance. As insulin resistance increases, so does the severity of hypertension.[32] Coconut oil, as you have learned in the discussion on diabetes, helps improve insulin sensitivity, making cells more responsive and less resistant and, therefore, helping protect against high blood pressure.

Studies of coconut eating populations show an absence of high blood pressure. In a study of two groups of Polynesians it was found that the group that consumed 89 percent of their fat as coconut oil had lower blood pressure values than those who ate only 7 percent.[33] In affluent countries blood pressure typically increases with age. In island populations where coconut is still a major

---

Blood Pressure

I put some virgin coconut oil in my tea in the morning where it melts. I then open a capsule with 100 mg CoQ10 and put the contents on top of the oil where they dissolve in the oil. Then I drink the tea as usual. This has lowered my blood pressure enormously so that I no longer need pills.

Hans

There is something to this coconut stuff, let me tell you…Had a 3-month check-up this morning…my blood pressure went from 210/142 to 134/77 and this after actually decreasing my blood pressure medicine!

Alice

A Physician's Story
By Marieta Jader-Onate, M.D.
Founder and CEO of the Good Shepherd Hospital
Lucena City, Philippines

I am 44 years old. I became a medical doctor in my mid 20's. My profession has been filled with a lot of excitement, dedication, and stress. Over the years I was too busy to eat, often skipped meals, and paid no attention to the types of foods I was eating.

Despite my poor eating habits and hectic lifestyle, my health held up well until I was 40, when I started to have elevated blood pressure associated with headaches and dizziness. I took antihypertensive drugs, which at first relieved my symptoms. After a month I began to have difficulty breathing and developed a fever accompanied by chest pain, joint pain, and numbness in my left leg. A CT scan was done, but showed no abnormalities. A 2-D echo revealed mitral valve prolapse, and lab results showed an elevated ASO titer (antistreptolysin O) elevated cholesterol level (LDL), and I was diagnosed as having hypertension and rheumatic fever with carditis.

A few months later severe abdominal pain, indigestion, and constipation set in. An ultrasound of the whole abdomen showed cholecystitis and cholelithiasis (inflammation and multiple stones of the gall bladder). My gallbladder was removed. Surgical recovery was long and painful. I still had on and off elevated blood pressure, chest pain, occasional difficulty breathing, indigestion, and constipation.

Hoping to find help with my health problems I reviewed my medical books and researched the medical literature. I discovered that coconut-based diets had sustained populations for thousands of years in apparent good health and that recent research indicated many health benefits from eating coconut, particularly coconut oil. I made a careful plan of my diet, and included mostly coconut products with my meals. I also took 1 tablespoon of virgin coconut oil three times a day. Sometimes I swallowed it directly followed by a glass of water, or I put it in my rice.

After changing to a coconut-based diet, I noted that my blood pressure became stable, and I had no chest pain, difficulty of breathing, indigestion, or constipation. My energy level was boosted. These amazing results prompted me to read more about the medical benefits of virgin coconut oil, and I started introducing it to my patients with excellent results.

part of the diet, blood pressure does not increase significantly with age.[34] Blood pressure remains at a healthy level throughout life even when they reach ages of 80 and 90 years.

From this discussion we can conclude that coconut oil does not contribute to high blood pressure and in many situations may help lower it, thus reducing risk of heart disease.

Homocysteine Levels

In recent years elevated blood levels of homocysteine (a sulfur-containing amino acid) has been gaining recognition as an important new risk factor in heart disease. It has been linked to increased risk of heart disease and stroke even among people who have normal cholesterol levels. Elevated homocysteine levels appear to damage cells lining the inside of the arteries. Studies indicate that elevated blood homocysteine levels are more accurate in predicting heart disease than high cholesterol, high blood pressure, and cigarette smoking. A review of all published studies on homocysteine indicates that it is one of, if not the most significant, independent risk factors for atherosclerosis. For every 10 percent elevation of homocysteine, there is a corresponding rise in the risk of developing severe coronary heart disease.[35]

The connection between homocysteine and cardiovascular disease was first suspected about 30 years ago when it was observed that people with a rare genetic condition called homocystinuria were prone to develop severe cardiovascular disease. One of the first reported cases involved an 8-year-old who exhibited all the signs of advanced atherosclerotic disease and died of a stroke—a curious death for someone so young. Atherosclerosis and stroke are considered diseases of aging.

Homocysteine is an amino acid derived from the metabolic breakdown of methionine—one of the essential amino acids obtained from protein in our food. It is particularly abundant in meat. When we eat protein-rich foods, methionine is converted into homocysteine. The liver converts homocysteine back into methionine or into other substances, so the concentration is normally kept very low. In homocystinuria, a genetic defect in the liver prevents the formation of enzymes that are necessary for homocysteine metabolization and, consequently, homocysteine concentrations build up in the body. The problem with homocysteine is that it is toxic to the arteries. A high blood level of homocysteine both initiates and accelerates atherosclerosis.

The enzymes that metabolize homocysteine are dependent on vitamins B-6, B-12, and folic acid. Abnormal elevation of homocysteine can occur in anyone whose diet contains inadequate amounts of these vitamins. A combination of a diet high in animal protein (a source of methionine and homocysteine) and low in B vitamins leads to elevated homocysteine levels. Our modern diet is high in animal protein and low in the foods that supply good

119

sources of B vitamins (fresh fruits, vegetables, and whole grains). Processed packaged foods, refined flour products, and sweets are sadly deficient in B vitamins.

Eating more fresh fruits, vegetables and whole grains, and reducing the amount of meat and processed foods you eat can lower your risk of heart disease by lowering homocysteine levels. Taking a dietary supplement that supplies the B vitamins has also shown to be useful in lowering homocysteine levels.

Using coconut oil daily can be of benefit too. When coconut oil is eaten with foods, it slows down the rate at which the stomach empties. This allows foods to remain in contact with digestive enzymes and stomach acids longer, thus increasing the amount of nutrients, including B vitamins that are released from the food. Coconut oil also enhances the rate at which many vitamins and minerals are absorbed. For these reasons, coconut oil has been recommended for the use in treating malnutrition. Excessive homocysteine in the blood is caused by a vitamin deficiency and is essentially a form of malnutrition. Coconut oil can help correct this condition and, in so doing, reduce the risk of heart disease.

Arterial Inflammation

A new heart disease risk factor has emerged in recent years that appears to be a better indicator of risk than any of the others. This new risk factor is chronic inflammation in the arteries. Chronic inflammation injures tissues, causing the development of arterial plaque and atherosclerosis. While most other risk factors only indicate an association with heart disease, arterial inflammation may be actively involved in its cause. The relationship between chronic arterial inflammation and heart disease is a much better indicator of heart disease risk than cholesterol.[36]

Arterial inflammation can be determined by measuring a substance in the blood called C-reactive protein (CRP). Dr. Paul Ridker of Brigham and Women's Hospital in Boston evaluated blood samples from more than 28,000 healthy nurses. Those with the highest levels of C-reactive protein had more than four times the risk of having heart trouble. He says, "We were able to find that the C-reactive protein is a stronger predictor of risk than were the regular cholesterol levels, and that's very important because almost half of all heart attacks occur among people who have normal cholesterol levels."

Inflammation of the arteries may explain heart disease in people without other known risk factors—people with normal cholesterol and low blood pressure who are non-diabetic and in good physical shape. These patients make up a third of all heart attack cases. Researchers have known for years that other factors must be involved in coronary artery disease.

What causes arteries to become inflamed? Although there may be several factors, the three primary ones associated with heart disease are 1) homocysteine levels, 2) oxidative stress, and 3) chronic low-grade infection. A high level of homocysteine in the blood is toxic to arterial tissues and causes injuries that lead to inflammation. This topic was discussed in some detail above. Let me talk about the other two.

Oxidative Stress

Oxidative stress occurs when the body contains insufficient antioxidants to adequately fend off the free radicals being generated. The destructive nature of free radicals was discussed in Chapter 3. Oxidative stress is believed to be important in the development of coronary artery disease because free-radical damaged lipids (fat and cholesterol) can become toxic and injure the heart and artery walls.

LDL cholesterol, which is produced by the body in the liver is harmless, and actually beneficial because the body uses it as building material for cell walls, to make vitamin D, and to synthesize many vital hormones. LDL cholesterol is known as the "bad" cholesterol because it is associated with arterial plaque. It only turns bad when it becomes oxidized. Oxidized cholesterol damages artery walls. Unoxidized cholesterol doesn't. Oxidized triglycerides (fats) also damage artery walls. In fact, oxidized fat and oxidized cholesterol are the only lipids found in arterial plaque. Unoxidized lipids don't go there.

Unsaturated fats (polyunsaturated and monounsaturated) are highly vulnerable to oxidation. When fats are exposed to heat, light, or oxygen for a period of time, they can become rancid and create free radicals. Oxidized fats are rancid fats. Fats can become rancid both inside and outside of the body. Some fats in your body are going rancid right now. It's part of the metabolic process. The only thing that keeps all of the unsaturated fats and cholesterol in our bodies from becoming oxidized is antioxidants. Antioxidants block the destructive action of free radicals and stops the oxidation process. When people are exposed to high levels of pollutants which act as pro-oxidants and don't eat enough fresh fruits and vegetables rich in antioxidants, the antioxidant reserves in the body become depleted. The rate at which fats and cholesterol are transformed into destructive artery-damaging fats is increased.

Increasing the amount of antioxidants in the diet can provide increased protection from oxidation. Diets rich in antioxidant vitamins have been specifically recommended for patients with heart disease.[37]

The benefit of coconut oil is that it is composed of 92 percent saturated fat, most of which is made of MCFAs. These fats are very stable and highly resistant to oxidation. So resistant, in fact, that they act as antioxidants. Like other antioxidants, MCFAs can protect unsaturated fats and cholesterol from oxidizing. Coconut oil helps reduce oxidative stress and thus helps protect against heart disease.

Ironically, saturated fat phobics have attempted to demonize coconut oil by labeling it an "artery clogging" fat. Coconut oil, however, does not clog up the arteries, but polyunsaturated fats do. Analysis of arterial plaque by Felton and colleagues show that oxidized fatty acids in arterial plaque are primarily *un*saturated, not saturated.[38] In fact, 74 percent of the fatty acids in arterial plaque are unsaturated (41 percent polyunsaturated and 33 percent monounsaturated). Not a single medium-chain fatty acid was found in the plaque. In truth, unsaturated fats, and particularly polyunsaturated fats, are the real artery-clogging fats.

Chronic Infection

Low-grade chronic infection is the third factor on our list. Low-grade infections can be caused by any number of pathogenic (disease-causing) bacteria or viruses. Some of these microorganisms can live in the body indefinitely. Once you've been infected by chickenpox, for instance, the virus remains with you for life, hiding out in the nervous system. If the immune system becomes stressed or weakened, the virus is able to multiply and reinfect the body. This time it expresses itself in the form of shingles—a common illness of the elderly. If pathogenic microorganisms find entry into the circulatory system they can infect artery walls, causing localized low-grade infections and chronic inflammation. In this manner, bacteria and viruses can conceivably cause atherosclerosis and heart disease.

Some years ago the Finnish government sponsored a comprehensive study of health risks. They measured the rates of numerous diseases and did statistical analysis to see if there were any correlations between them. Unexpectedly they found a link between dental disease and heart disease. Those people who had periodontal or gum disease had a significantly higher incidence of heart disease. Additional studies in the United States and Europe confirmed the results. These studies found that people with periodontal disease had a 200 percent higher risk of dying from cardiovascular disease.[39] By comparison, smokers only have a 60 percent increased risk. The presence of periodontal disease is a far more accurate indicator of heart disease risk than smoking. Oral health parameters such as dental plaque, cavities, and gum disease have now become recognized as being more strongly associated with coronary heart disease than recognized standard risk factors such as blood cholesterol levels, being overweight, diabetes, not exercising, and smoking status.[40]

Periodontal disease is caused by a chronic bacterial infection in the mouth. If the immune system is incapable of adequately controlling the infection, it can spread into the bloodstream and affect the arteries. People with periodontal disease also have high levels of C-reactive protein—the indicator of arterial inflammation. Dr. Efthymios Deliargyris, and others at the University of North Carolina at Chapel Hill studied 38 heart attack sufferers and found that 85 percent of them had chronic periodontitis and high levels of C-reactive protein. In comparison only 29 percent of healthy volunteers had these conditions.

Since the initial studies with periodontal disease, other infectious conditions have been linked with heart disease. Research suggests that sinusitis, bronchitis, stomach ulcers, herpes, and urinary tract infections could also play a role in heart disease.[41] The three most prevalent organisms associated with arterial inflammation are *Helicobacter pylori, Chlamydia pneumoniae,* and cytomegalovirus (CMV). *Helicobacter pylori* is a bacterium that is the primary cause of stomach ulcers. *Chlamydia pneumoniae,* another bacterium, causes periodontal disease, conjunctivitis, and pneumonia. CMV is an extremely common herpes virus. Approximately 80 percent of adults have antibodies to it in their blood, which is an indication of a past or present infection. Symptoms are generally so mild that the infection goes unnoticed.

Bacteria and viruses that cause these infections can find their way into the circulatory system. If the immune system is incapable of adequately controlling these organisms, they can embed themselves into the artery walls, causing a chronic low-grade infection. The infection irritates surrounding tissues, which causes inflammation and, consequently, the development of atherosclerosis. The connection between infections and atherosclerosis is strengthened by the fact that fragments of bacteria are often found inside arterial plaque. Brent Muhlestein, a cardiologist at the LDS Hospital in Salt Lake City and the University of Utah has found the 79 percent of plaque specimens taken from the coronary arteries of 90 heart disease patients contained evidence of chlamydia.

Because of the strong evidence linking chronic low-grade infections to heart disease, antibiotics have been suggested as a means for treatment. The problem with this approach, however, is that not all low-grade infections are caused by bacteria. Antibiotics are only good against bacteria. They don't do a thing to viruses. The overuse of antibiotics has caused a new problem with bacteria developing resistance to antibiotics. So antibiotics aren't the answer.

What role does coconut oil have in all of this? As you learned in Chapter 3, MCFAs possess powerful antimicrobial properties capable of destroying disease-causing bacteria and viruses. It just so happens that the primary culprits linked to arterial inflammation: *H. pylori,* Chlamydia, and CMV are all killed by MCFAs. Medium-chain fatty acids can rid the body of these troublesome organisms without harming friendly gut bacteria or promoting antibiotic resistance. Antibiotics can't do this. At this point no drug or medical procedure can safely and effectively kill all the microorganisms involved in arterial inflammation. Research has shown that arterial inflammation is the strongest risk factor associated with heart disease. Reducing this risk will do more to prevent heart disease than anything else you can do, including taking cholesterol-lowering drugs.

All you need to do is add coconut oil to your daily diet. Since MCFAs in coconut oil kill the organisms that cause arterial inflammation, coconut oil reduces the risk of heart disease.

Other Risk Factors

The risk factors for heart disease listed above are the most universally recognized. Researchers have identified other possible risk factors that are influenced by diet and lifestyle. These include the following:

Vitamin E deficiency
Vitamin C deficiency
Selenium deficiency
Magnesium deficiency
Protein deficiency
Excess sugar consumption
Hypothyroidism

We need a continual supply of antioxidants in our diet to protect us from the destructive action of free radicals. A deficiency of antioxidant vitamins and minerals such as vitamins E and C and the mineral selenium can lead to oxidative stress, which promotes heart disease. When antioxidants fend off free radicals, they are consumed and our antioxidant defenses decline. Coconut oil also acts as a protective antioxidant, blocking free radical reactions. In this way it spares other antioxidants from being destroyed and helps prevent deficiencies of these important nutrients.

In addition to protecting antioxidants from free radicals, coconut oil has shown to improve the absorption of many nutrients in our food. In this way it helps to protect against deficiencies of vitamin E, vitamin C, selenium, magnesium, and protein.

Sugar and refined carbohydrates have an adverse effect on blood sugar and insulin levels. Excess consumption of these products has been suggested as contributing factors to various health problems including diabetes, metabolic syndrome, and heart disease. Coconut oil dampens the effects of sugar and starch on blood glucose and insulin levels, thus helping protect against these problems.

Evidence suggests that low thyroid function contributes to heart disease. Thyroid dysfunction doesn't even have to be severe in order to affect the heart. In one study, for example, it was found the heart disease developed 2.6 times more frequently in those who had subclinical hypothyroidism than those with normal thyroid function.[42] One of the symptoms of hypothyroidism is low body temperature due to a drop in metabolism. Many of the enzymes in the body that govern chemical processes are highly sensitive to temperature variations. When body temperatures are below normal, these enzymes slow down. Vital chemical processes in the body consequently slow down as well. This leads to abnormal fat metabolism. Combined with a reduced ability to heal and repair itself due to sub-normal metabolism, arteries are more prone to accumulate plaque.

Again coconut comes to the rescue. Coconut oil speeds up metabolism and increases body temperature. This allows temperature-dependent enzymes and healing to function at a more normal level.

Vitamin, mineral, and protein deficiencies, excess sugar consumption, and hypothyroidism—in each case coconut oil reduces the risk of heart disease.

The more risk factors you have, the higher the probability or risk of developing heart disease. Anything that would increase any one of the risk factors mentioned in this chapter is considered undesirable because it has the potential to increase your risk of suffering a heart attack or stroke. Anything that would reduce these risk factors would be considered protective against heart disease.

After reviewing all the risk factors for heart disease discussed in this chapter, how many are negatively influenced by the consumption of coconut oil? The answer is "none." That's right, not a single one of these risk factors are negatively influenced by coconut oil. Coconut oil has a *positive* effect on *all* of these risk factors. For this reason, coconut oil consumption should be considered a means to reduce risk and protect against heart disease.

Few, if any, other procedures or substances currently recommended for the prevention of heart disease have such a positive effect on so many risk factors. Polyunsaturated oils are considered protective against heart disease simply because they reduce just one of these factors—total blood cholesterol. Taking B vitamins are considered protective because they help reduce homocysteine levels. Cholesterol-lowering drugs, which are aggressively promoted as the primary means to prevent heart disease, don't even come close to comparing to coconut oil. While they do help to reduce total cholesterol, they don't necessarily improve the cholesterol ratio, a far more important risk indicator. They also don't do a thing to help with other risk factors such as diabetes, obesity, or homocysteine levels. Their side effects can even be harmful. They reduce antioxidant reserves in the body, thus increasing oxidative stress and can be toxic to the liver, kidneys, and muscle tissues. In contrast, coconut oil is harmless. It has no known detrimental side effects. It is a food that nourishes the body.

If coconut oil were a drug developed in some laboratory, the pharmaceutical industry would have it advertised all over the place as the best thing there is for heart disease protection. It would be spotlighted in newspaper and magazine articles and be a hot topic on all the popular radio and television talk shows. And what would they charge for it? A month's supply would probably cost you two weeks pay and your left leg.

Fortunately, coconut oil is not a drug, does not cost an arm and a leg, and is available and safe for all to use. If you are concerned about heart disease, coconut oil is one of the best things you can use to prevent it.

Chapter 6

COCONUT MEDICINE CHEST II: COCONUT MEAT, WATER, AND MILK

In this chapter, we cover the second portion of The Coconut Medicine Chest. The health aspects of coconut meat, water, and milk are described. Although much of the health benefits of these products come from the fat or oil they contain, each product has its own unique advantages.

COCONUT MEAT

Coconut has been called the "king of foods." It is used as both a food to sustain life and as a medicine to restore health. Tradition has it that eating the fruit of the coconut tree is one of the secrets to good health and a long life. No other single food, to my knowledge, offers as much healthwise as the coconut. Indeed, many people have lived for extended periods of time with little more than coconuts to sustain them. Some island populations thrive on a diet consisting predominately of coconut. For generations they have lived without the sickness and disease that plagues modern society. Few, if any, other foods could as adequately provide for both the nutritional and medicinal needs of the human body. The coconut is truly the king of foods.

The meat from a fully matured coconut is hard, white, and slightly sweet with a nutty flavor. In the tropics immature coconuts—also called green or young coconuts—are a delicacy. The meat is only partially developed and has a gelatinous texture. It is soft enough that you can eat it with a spoon and tastes distinctly different from the meat of a mature coconut. The soft meat from a young coconut is often given to babies as their first food during weaning. As the coconut ages, the meat thickens and hardens. Young coconuts spoil much quicker than mature nuts so they are less often found at the market outside the tropics. If you do find them in temperate climates, they are kept cool to prevent spoiling. As the coconut matures, the oil and fiber content increases.

A Functional Food

Like the oil, coconut meat is clearly a functional food. It provides many health benefits beyond its nutritional content. The meat from a mature coconut contains all the nutritional and health benefits associated with the oil discussed in the previous chapters. That means it improves digestion and nutritional status, protects against cancer and heart disease, aids in weight loss, kills disease-causing microorganisms and parasites, as well as all the other benefits associated with the oil. The reason for this is that coconut meat contains a high amount of oil. It is from the meat that coconut oil is extracted. Coconut meat by weight consists of 34 percent oil. That's a large percentage of oil and the reason why it is so easily extracted from the meat.

Fresh coconut meat by weight is 47 percent water. When the meat is dried, the water content is reduced to about 3 percent. Without the water, the proportion of fat increases; dried coconut contains 64 percent fat. Eating both fresh and dried coconut provides a good source of this health promoting oil.

COMPOSITON OF COCONUT		
(% by weight)		
	Fresh	**Dried**
Water	47	3
Fat	34	64
Fiber	11	15
Protein	4	9
Starch and Sugar	4	9

Other than water, the two main ingredients in coconut are fat and fiber. The fiber content is important because it provides benefits beyond that of just the oil.

There are two types of carbohydrate in foods: digestible and non-digestible. Digestible carbohydrate consists of starch and sugar and provides calories. Non-digestible carbohydrate is simply dietary fiber and since it is not broken down or digested in humans, it provides no calories.

Coconut contains very little digestible carbohydrate, making it an excellent choice for those people looking for low carbohydrate foods. One cup of shredded *fresh* coconut (80 grams) contains a mere 3 grams of digestible carbohydrate and 9 grams of fiber. Dried coconut has a slightly higher digestible carbohydrate content; 1 cup of shredded dried coconut contains 7 grams of digestible carbohydrate and 12 grams of fiber. Coconut is a great way to add bulk and flavor to foods without adding too many calories from carbohydrate.

Fresh coconut contains a total of 15 percent carbohydrate—4 percent digestible and 11 percent non-digestible. The rest (85 percent) is composed primarily of water, fat, and protein. It contains far more non-digestible (fiber) carbohydrate than it does digestible carbohydrate, making it an excellent source of dietary fiber. In fact, it is by far one of the most concentrated sources of dietary fiber. According to the U.S. Department of Agriculture, 24 percent of the carbohydrate in oat bran is composed of fiber. Wheat bran is 42 percent fiber. Soybeans contain only 29 percent fiber. Coconut beats them all. Its carbohydrate content is composed of a whopping 71 percent fiber!

Next to sawdust, wheat bran is one of the highest sources of fiber you can find. Coconut contains almost twice as much fiber as wheat bran and unlike bran, it doesn't taste like cardboard. Coconut is one source of fiber that

Fiber in Carbohydrate Portion of Foods

The carbohydrate in foods is composed of both digestible carbohydrate (starch and sugar) and non-digestible carbohydrate (fiber). The amount of each varies with each food. The list below shows the amount of fiber in select foods as a percentage of total carbohydrate content. For example, 71 percent of the total carbohydrate content in fresh coconut is from fiber. The remaining 29 percent is composed of starch and sugar.

Nuts
Coconut (fresh) 71
Almonds 56
Peanuts 48
Hazelnuts 39
Pecans 35
Walnuts 32
Cashews 18

Vegetables
Bamboo Shoots 75
Broccoli 60
Spinach 57
Zucchini 57
Cabbage 50
Cauliflower 50
Red Radish 50
Mushrooms 50

Kidney Beans 49
Lima beans 46
Pinto Beans 45
Green Peas 36
Asparagus 33
Okra 33
Tomato 33
Kelp 33
Green Beans 30
Beets 29
Soybeans 29
Carrots 29
Butternut Squash 27
Lentils 25
Garbanzo 24
Onion 21
Bell Pepper 20
Acorn Squash 19

Sweet Potato 11
Potato (with skin) 10

Fruits
Strawberries 36
Kiwi 27
Grapefruit 22
Mango 20
Orange 20
Peach 20
Apple 14
Papaya 14
Grapes 11
Pineapple 11
Plum 11
Cherries 9
Banana 7
Watermelon 6

actually tastes good. If you want to add more fiber to your diet, coconut is an excellent way to go.

Nutritionists recommend that we get between 20 to 35 grams of fiber a day. This is 2 to 3 times higher than the average daily intake in Western diets, which is about 10 to 14 grams. One cup of dried shredded coconut (unpacked) contains 12 grams of fiber. One small 2 x 2-inch piece of fresh coconut contains 5 grams of fiber. Adding fresh or dried coconut to your diet can significantly improve your daily fiber intake.

Why Fiber is Good For You

Imagine for a moment a food, a superfood, that can satisfy your appetite, has virtually no calories, can lower cholesterol and blood sugar, and can reduce your risk of heart disease, high blood pressure, diabetes, and intestinal diseases like irritable bowel syndrome and colon cancer. Most foods or dietary supplements that are supposed to provide a multitude of health benefits generally taste awful. Have you ever tasted cod liver oil? How about wheat bran? Yuck. That's how my kids describe these "health" foods. Suppose this superfood has a mild, delightful taste that you and your family would enjoy eating. Would you be interested in adding this food into your diet? Who wouldn't?

You hear a lot about the need for fiber these days. Yet, not too long ago fiber was considered a non-nutrient—an inconsequential part of the diet. Fiber is found in all plant foods. It is that portion of the plant that cannot be digested by enzymes in the human digestive tract. Because fiber is not digested, it does not provide nutrients or supply any calories. For this reason, it was thought to be unimportant to health. We now know that fiber plays a significant role in the digestive process and can dramatically affect our state of health. Although fiber does not supply calories or building blocks for the body, it is now considered an essential nutrient. A deficiency of fiber in the diet leads to many health problems. For this reason, it is just as important as vitamin C or calcium or any other essential nutrient.

The importance of fiber in our diet was first noted by physicians working in Africa, India, and Oceania in the early and mid-twentieth century. They observed that people eating traditional diets, which were high in fiber, enjoyed a level of health better than those in Western countries. Absent were the health problems commonly seen in Europe and America. However, when these people began eating Western foods, rich in refined grains and sugar, their health deteriorated and they developed many of same health problems commonly found in Western countries.

Physicians noticed that in rural communities where fiber intake was high, degenerative disease was low. Where fiber consumption was low, due to the use of modern foods, disease rates were much higher. This observation led to what is known as the "fiber hypothesis" which suggests that the consumption of unrefined, high-fiber foods protect against many degenerative health problems common in Western countries.

One of the leading proponents of the fiber hypothesis was British surgeon and epidemiologist Denis Burkitt, MD. His research was primarily responsible for changing the image of dietary fiber from that of a useless bystander to that of an active player in the promotion and maintenance of good health.

Working in rural Africa in the mid-1900s Burkitt observed that the bowel habits of rural Africans were very different from those of the British. Africans passed soft, odorless stools four times the weight of the British, which in comparison were small, dry, and smelly. They noted that in Africans, food traveled through their digestive tracts and was expelled in as little as one day, compared to a full three or more days for the British. The Africans' diet consisted primarily of high-fiber foods such as cereals, beans, peas, and root vegetables like potatoes and yams. In contrast, the British diet was composed predominately of white flour products, high in sugar and meat. The researchers calculated that Africans consumed between 60-120 grams of fiber a day, while the British consumed only about a fifth this much. The Africans' high-fiber diet obviously accounted for their large, soft, frequent bowel movements. The significance of their bowel habits was recognized when it was observed that many of the digestive problems common in Britain were completely absent among the African villagers. Not only were there fewer digestive problems, but they were also free from most all other non-infectious diseases as well, and none of them were overweight. Dietary fiber, it was reasoned, must have some connection to overall health beyond just bowel function.

It quickly became apparent that the most striking consequence of not having enough fiber in the diet was constipation. Based on his studies in Africa and elsewhere Burkitt drew a direct connection between constipation and five other common health problems: diverticular disease, appendicitis, hiatal hernia, hemorrhoids, and varicose veins. Each of these, he said, was caused by straining to expel hard fecal matter.

Fiber is important because it regulates bowel activity. It absorbs water, providing a medium that is moist and mobile which can speedily sweep the inside of the bowel clean. Fiber, in essence, is nature's way of keeping our intestines clean, healthy, and functioning smoothly.

Fecal bulk is more than just fiber and undigested food. It also contains bacteria, intestinal secretions, and the remains of dead intestinal cells. Bacteria make up the largest percentage of the fecal mass—about a third.

Digestion starts in the mouth, continues in the stomach, and finishes off in the small and large intestines. Along the way food is mixed with liquids and enzymes to assist in breaking it down and transporting it through the digestive tract. The majority of digestion and assimilation takes place during the meandrous 20-foot journey through the small intestine. As food travels along the small intestine, nutrients are released and absorbed into the bloodstream. By the time it reaches the end of the small intestine most of the nutrients have been extracted, leaving indigestible fiber, dead cells, and other debris. This waste material then enters the large intestine. Although this portion of the digestive tract is much shorter than the small intestine—being only about five feet in length—it is a good deal wider, thus it is called the *large* intestine. It is also known as the colon or bowel.

In the colon, waste material (called feces or stool) is prepared for elimination. When this material enters the colon it is very liquid, like a soup. One of the functions of the colon is to extract fluid from the waste to make it more compact and semi-solid. As the feces travel through the colon, water is gradually absorbed, producing a mass that is more solid, yet still soft enough to be excreted with ease. Undigested fiber provides bulk and body to the feces, allowing intestinal muscles to easily and quickly move the mass along its path and out of the body without interruption.

As the amount of dietary fiber decreases, transit time through the colon slows down. The longer this material remains in the colon, the more fluid is extracted and the feces becomes harder and more difficult for the muscles to move through the colon. The harder it gets, the slower it moves, and the longer the transit time, leading to even more fluid extraction and slower transit time. A vicious cycle is created and constipation results. When little dietary fiber is present, fecal material can become hardened and impacted. Bowel evacuations become arduous chores involving prolonged straining. Stools are hard, dry, and infrequent.

A diet low in fiber and, consequently, high in refined, overly processed foods leads to constipation, which in turn, can set the stage for a number of health problems. Excessive pressures caused by hardened fecal material can damage tissues within the colon. Pressures can become so great trying to move this hardened mass through the colon that tissues in the intestinal wall break down, give way, and begin to bulge, sometimes forming pockets that fill with hardened waste. These pockets of fecal waste are called diverticula. People can have literally dozens of diverticula ranging in size from a fingertip to a tennis ball. A person who has many of them is said to have diverticular disease or diverticulosis. Once diverticula form, there is no way to get rid of them save surgery. As long as they don't become inflamed or infected, they are generally left alone. After the age of 40 one half of all Americans develop diverticular disease. In his 20 years working in Africa Dr. Burkitt did not see a single case of diverticular disease.

High pressure caused by the sluggish movement of waste can weaken and deform the colon, causing bulging, stretching, and tears in the lining of the bowel. These conditions can lead not only to diverticulosis but also to appendicitis, hemorrhoids, hiatal hernia, varicose veins, prolapsed colon, heartburn, even gallstones, and may contribute to ulcerative colitis and Crohn's disease.

Dr. Burkitt says that when he first went to Africa he worked in a 600-bed teaching hospital. They wouldn't see more than two patients with appendicitis in an entire year. In comparison, a hospital of the same size in the United States would have two cases of appendicitis a day! When African soldiers joined British troops in North Africa during the Second World War and began eating British soldiers' rations, they began for the first time to get appendicitis. Those who get appendicitis in Africa now are the educated people who have taken on Western eating habits.

Burkitt says, "We used to teach our students never to diagnose appendicitis in an African patient, no matter what the clinical symptoms, unless the patient could speak English. Nobody gets appendicitis until after they learn English in East Africa. Speaking English is an index of an African's contact with modern Western culture."

Hiatal hernia is a condition in which the stomach is pushed upward out of the abdominal cavity and into the thoracic cavity. When the muscles of the abdominal wall contract to assist in the evacuation of a constipated stool, pressure within the abdomen is increased, and as a result, the upper end of the stomach is squeezed up out of the abdomen into the thorax. A common symptom is heartburn. In fact, frequent heartburn is an indication of excessive abdominal pressure. In North America one adult in four is affected by hiatal hernia. A radiological study in West Africa reported by Burkitt found only one case in over 1,000 patients in Kenya and one in over 700 cases in Tanzania.[1]

Hemorrhoids and varicose veins are also caused by constipation and excessive abdominal pressure. About half the American population experiences hemorrhoids. At least 50 percent of American women over the age of 40 have varicose veins. These conditions, common in affluent societies, are uncommon in other parts of the world where dietary fiber consumption is higher. A study in Papua New Guinea examined 800 adult women and found only one with a small varicose vein. It is believed that the straining due to constipation can cause blood to be forced to flow back down the legs, causing the valves to stretch. Eventually, the veins will not be able to function properly, and varicose veins develop.

Gallstones are one of the most common complaints of women. About one woman in three in North America eventually develops gallstones. In Africa, Burkitt found there were virtually no gallstones. Only twice in a 20-year surgical practice did Burkitt remove a gallbladder from an African woman. Excessive pressure may again be the underlying cause by interfering with the flow of bile, which contributes to gallstone formation.

Since the fiber hypothesis was first proposed, a host of other conditions characteristic of modern Western civilization have been shown to be related to intestinal transit time (the amount of time it takes food to pass through the digestive tract). As researchers began to study the relationship between dietary fiber and health, one notable effect stood out. It didn't matter if a man or a woman lived in a little rural village in Africa or on the 30th floor of a skyscraper in New York City, if their diet was high in fiber, they were spared from many of the health problems common in our society, including one of the scourges of modern civilization—obesity.

The lack of adequate fiber in the diet is believed to be responsible for a variety of health problems. Research suggest that dietary fiber can help prevent and treat:

Obesity	High cholesterol
Constipation and diarrhea	High blood pressure
Hemorrhoids	Hypoglycemia (low blood sugar)
Appendicitis	Diabetes
Diverticulosis	Colon cancer
Varicose veins	Breast cancer
Hiatal hernia	Prostate cancer
Gallstones	Ovarian cancer
Irritable bowel syndrome	Candidiasis
Colitis and Crohn's disease	Depression and irritability
Heartburn	Toxic accumulation
Heart disease and stroke	

Constipation and Intestinal Transit Time

Constipation is so prevalent nowadays that most people don't even know how to recognize it. Having a bowel movement every two or three days is considered normal. Even the medical profession has become so accustomed to seeing constipated people that they judge constipation by what is typical or average. Unfortunately, the average is not a good standard on which to judge when most everyone has the same problem. What's normal and what's healthy are two different things.

How can you tell if you're constipated? The best way to tell is to compare yourself with someone who has excellent digestive health, for example, rural Africans who eat a high-fiber diet and have optimal digestive function. They have a bowel movement for every meal they eat. If you eat three meals a day, you should have as many as three movements a day. In general, a healthy adult should have at least one and as many as three semi-solid (not runny) movements each day.

Feces should not be hard and elimination should be easy and brief. If not, you need to add more fiber into your diet and cut down on overly processed foods.

Another way to determine if you need to add more fiber to your diet is to measure the transit time of the foods you eat. Bowel transit time is the time it takes for food to travel completely through your digestive tract. To test yourself, all you need to do is to eat some food that normally isn't completely digested, such as fresh corn. This food serves as a marker. The starch in the corn is easily digested but the bran, which makes up the outer fibrous part of the kernel, isn't. It can be visible after a bowel movement. Simply eat some fresh corn or corn on the cob. Watch your eliminations and make note of when the kernels come through. A healthy transit time is 18 to 30 hours—no more and no less. In the United States and Europe bowel transit times are typically 2 to 3 days (48 to 60 hours). If it takes longer than 30 hours for the corn to pass through your body, you need more fiber in your diet. Likewise, if the corn kernels pass in less than 18 hours you may also have a problem. If foods travel through the digestive tract too rapidly, then nutrients are not properly digested and absorbed. This can lead to nutrient deficiencies. In this case, dietary fiber will help speed up transit time. So if your food passes through your digestive tract too quickly or too slowly, adding dietary fiber will moderate transit time.

Fiber and Cancer

The link between dietary fiber and cancer is most noticeable with colon cancer. Fiber acts like a broom, sweeping the intestinal contents through the digestive tract. Parasites, toxins, and carcinogens are swept along with the fiber, leading to their timely expulsion from the body. This cleansing action helps prevent toxins that irritate intestinal tissues and cause cancer from getting lodged in the intestinal tract. Colon cancer is second only to lung cancer as the world's most deadly form of cancer. Many studies have shown a correlation between high-fiber diets and a low incidence of colon cancer. For example, in one of the most extensive studies to date, involving over 400,000 people from nine European countries, it was found that those who had the highest fiber intake were 40 percent less likely to develop colon cancer.

Fiber readily absorbs fluids. It also appears to absorb harmful carcinogens and other toxic chemicals. Researchers at the University of Lund, Sweden, found that fiber in the diet can absorb substances such as quinolines that cause cancer. Quinolines are very potent carcinogens. Various types of fiber were examined for their absorption capacity and found to leach out up to 20 to 50 percent of these compounds.

Dr. B.H. Ershoff of Loma Linda University summarized studies reported by the Committee on Nutrition in Medical Education. Studies compared groups of rats and mice, some given high-fiber diets and others given low-fiber diets.

The animals were fed various drugs, chemicals, and food additives such as cyclamate. These substances proved to be poisonous to the animals on the low-fiber diets, yet those given high-fiber diets showed no deleterious effects.[2]

Logically you can see the relationship between dietary fiber and its protective effect in the colon, but studies also show it protects against breast, prostate, and ovarian cancers as well. One explanation for this is that toxins lingering in the colon are absorbed into the bloodstream, and the blood then carries these toxins to other parts of the body where they can cause cancer.

Another explanation involves estrogen. Estrogen is required for the early growth and development of breast and ovarian cancer. The liver collects estrogen and sends it into the intestines where it is reabsorbed into the bloodstream. A high-fiber diet interrupts this process. Less estrogen is allowed back into the bloodstream because the activities of bacterial enzymes in the intestine are reduced. Studies show that serum estrogen can be significantly reduced by a high-fiber diet. Progesterone, which is an antagonist to estrogen and helps protect against cancer, is not affected or reduced by fiber.[3]

One of the main reasons proposed to explain why dietary fiber protects against colon and other cancers is that it decreases intestinal transit time. If carcinogenic substances, hormones, and toxins are quickly moved through the digestive tract and out of the body, they don't get a chance of irritating tissues and instigating cancer. Coconut fiber not only absorbs and sweeps carcinogenic toxins out of the intestinal tract, it also helps prevent the conditions that promote cancer. Evidence suggests that coconut fiber may also prevent the formation of tumors in the colon by moderating the harmful effects of tumor-promoting enzymes.[4]

Intestinal Health

Although we do not get nourishment from fiber, it feeds friendly bacteria in our gut that are essential for good health. These bacteria produce vitamins and other substances that are beneficial in promoting health and wellness. When we eat adequate amounts of fiber, intestinal bacteria flourish. Harmful bacteria and yeast, such as candida, which compete for space in the intestinal tract, are kept under control.

One of the most important reasons why friendly bacteria are important to our health is that they produce short-chain fatty acids (SCFAs). Short-chain fatty acids are fats that are synthesized from dietary fiber by intestinal bacteria, and which are vital to our health and the health of the colon. SCFAs are very similar to the MCFAs found in coconut oil and possess many of the same characteristics. Like MCFAs, short-chain fatty acids have the ability to kill disease-causing microorganisms.[5] Although they are generally not as potent as MCFAs in killing microorganisms, their presence in the colon helps keep harmful bacteria and yeasts under control. Another similarity between SCFAs and MCFAs is their ability to pass through cell membranes and into the mitochondria without the aid of special hormones (insulin) or enzymes (carnitine). Therefore, they can easily enter the cells in the colon where they are utilized as fuel to power metabolism. SCFAs are an important source of nutrition for the cells in the colon. In fact, SCFAs are the preferred food of colonic cells.

SCFAs also make a significant impact on the environment within the colon. While these SCFAs are harmless to our tissues and friendly bacteria, they are deadly to many forms of disease-causing bacteria and yeasts that can infect the intestinal tract. SCFAs can kill these troublesome organisms. The benefits which intestinal bacteria provide us are dependent on the amount of fiber we feed them. The more fiber we eat, the more friendly bacteria will thrive and produce SCFAs, thus keeping our colon healthy and nasty microorganisms in check.

Researchers have discovered that an abnormally low level of SCFAs in the colon can lead to nutritional deficiencies, which can cause inflammation and bleeding. SCFAs administered rectally into the colon relieve these conditions.[6]

The fiber in coconut acts as food for gut bacteria. Consequently, coconut helps prevent and relieve symptoms associated with Crohn's disease, irritable bowel syndrome, colitis, and other digestive disorders. Many people have reported that even eating as little as two coconut macaroon cookies a day relieves their symptoms. A newspaper health column from King Features Syndicate included a letter from a reader who had an interesting experience involving coconut.

"More than 20 years ago I was diagnosed with irritable bowel syndrome (IBS). Tests revealed no cause. Diarrhea attacks accompanied by severe abdominal pain rarely gave me time to find a bathroom before it was too late. I would suffer several times a week. At 6 feet 2 inches tall I weighed only 147 pounds and could not gain weight, even eating 5,000 calories a day. Imodium A-D daily provided minimal help. Ten months ago I read in your column about a man with Crohn's disease who had been helped by eating two Archway Coconut Macaroons daily. I had nothing to lose, so I gave it a try. IT HAS CHANGED MY LIFE! In these past 10 months I have had only a few mild attacks, none involving pain. Even the worst of these was milder than a good day before. I stopped carrying a change of clothes in my car, as I haven't needed them once. Twenty years of suffering, and all I needed to do was eat cookies! There is not one medication on the market that can boast fewer side effects. My weight is now stable at 180 pounds, ideal for my height."

Sometime later another reader wrote in and stated, "I've read in your column about coconut macaroon cookies as a treatment for chronic diarrhea. My dog has been diagnosed with irritable bowel syndrome, for which he has been prescribed prednisone. I know you were suggesting the cookies for people, but I figured, why not for my dog? On two coconut macaroons a day and no prednisone, he is getting much better. I wish I had known about this approach for my mother who had Crohn's disease."

The author of the column added that she had received several letters from people who reported similar results from eating coconut alone and one man reported that coconut-containing candy bars (Mounds) helped his antibiotic-induced diarrhea. Eating two coconut cookies or a candy bar a day—what a pleasant and easy way to stop the pain and discomfort caused by IBS and other gastrointestinal disorders. I don't personally recommend eating cookies and candy bars; there are better ways to eat coconut without all the sugar. The best way is to simply eat a piece of fresh coconut.

Weight Management

Since we cannot digest dietary fiber, we do not derive any calories from it. Dietary fiber is calorie-free. You can eat as much as you like without worrying about gaining weight—good news for those who are concerned about their weight.

Fiber absorbs water like a sponge. For this reason it aids in filling the stomach and producing a feeling of fullness. It provides bulk without supplying fat-promoting calories. Fiber also slows down the emptying of the stomach, thus maintaining the feeling of fullness longer than low-fiber foods. As a result, less food and fewer calories are consumed.

Studies have shown that consumption of an additional 14 grams of fiber a day (the amount in about ½ cup of coconut flour) is associated with a 10 percent decrease in calorie intake and a loss in body weight. The observed changes occur both when the fiber is from naturally high-fiber foods, like grains, beans, or coconut, and when it is from a fiber supplement, like wheat bran or coconut dietary fiber or flour.

When you eat high-fiber foods, which are generally low in calories, you crowd out higher calorie foods. Simply adding high-fiber foods into your diet will lower your calorie intake even if you eat the same volume of food you normally do. This fact was demonstrated by a study in which a group of overweight men were asked to eat 12 slices of whole wheat bread each day in addition to whatever other foods they wanted to eat. They could eat any other food they desired—desserts, fatty meats, cream—it didn't matter as long as it was food they normally ate. The study lasted for three months. At the end of the study the volunteers lost an average of 19.4 pounds. As long as they consumed the required amount of whole wheat bread, they were allowed to eat as much as they wanted. The bread was so filling that they didn't want a lot of other foods.[7]

Studies have shown that populations that rely heavily on coconut do not have weight problems. In one study, for example, an island population of 203 individuals ages 20 to 86 were examined. Researchers noted that they were all lean despite an abundance of food.[8] These people ate as much as they wanted, but overweight problems did not exist because their diet was rich in fiber, particularly from coconut.

Blood Sugar and Diabetes

Fiber is beneficial for diabetics and anyone else with blood sugar problems. When carbohydrates (starch and sugar) are eaten, they are quickly converted into glucose and pumped into the bloodstream. This creates a rapid rise in blood sugar (glucose). Insulin is needed to transfer glucose from the blood and into the cells. If blood sugar levels rise too high or remain elevated for too long it can cause numerous health problems. This is the situation that occurs in diabetics. Their bodies don't produce enough insulin to keep blood sugar levels under control. Any jump in blood sugar can be dangerous. This is why they must carefully watch what foods they eat, monitor their blood sugar levels, and take insulin injections as needed. In non-diabetics blood sugar levels are more quickly rebalanced so problems are less likely.

Fiber helps regulate blood sugar by slowing down the conversion of complex carbohydrates into sugar. Sugars are released at a slower rate and enter the bloodstream in smaller amounts. This keeps blood sugar and insulin levels under control.

Drs. Anderson and Gustafson of the University of Kentucky and the Endocrine-Metabolic Section of the Veterans Administration Medical Center in Lexington reported that a high-fiber diet helps reduce the need for insulin to the extent that fiber eliminates the need for insulin injections for two-thirds of patients who developed diabetes in later years. They went on to report that a high-fiber diet cut back by 25 percent the amount of insulin needed by diabetics whose diabetes began in childhood.[9]

Coconut fiber has been shown to be very effective in moderating blood sugar and insulin levels.[10] For this reason, coconut is good for diabetics. Diabetics are encouraged to eat foods that have a relatively low glycemic index. The glycemic index is a measure of how foods affect blood sugar levels. The higher the glycemic index value, the greater an effect a particular food has on raising blood sugar. So diabetics need to eat foods with a low glycemic index. When coconut is added to foods, including those high in starch and sugar, it *lowers* the glycemic index of these foods. This was clearly demonstrated by T. P. Trinidad and colleagues.[11] In their study, both normal and diabetic subjects were given a variety of foods to eat. Some of the types of food included cinnamon bread, granola bars, carrot cake, macaroons, and brownies—all foods that a diabetic must ordinarily limit because of their high sugar and starch content. It was found that as the coconut content of the foods increased, the blood sugar response between the diabetic and non-diabetic subjects became nearly identical. In other words, coconut moderated the release of sugar into the bloodstream so that there was no spike in blood glucose levels. As the coconut content in the foods decreased, the diabetic subjects' blood sugar levels became elevated, as would normally be expected from eating foods high in sugar and white flour. This study showed that adding coconut to foods lowers the glycemic index of the foods and keeps blood sugar levels under control.

Before Western foods were routinely shipped to the islands of the Pacific, diabetes was unheard of there. These people lived on a coconut-based diet with lots of sweet fruits and starchy vegetables. Only after they began to take on Western eating habits, low in fiber, did diabetes appear.

There is a little island in the Pacific called Nauru. It is only 12 miles around. The people lived for centuries on coconut and other produce that grew on the island. Diabetes was nonexistent. In 1952 they discovered a rich market for the huge phosphate deposits on the island. The phosphates, which are used in fertilizer, came from bird droppings that had been accumulating on the island for long periods of time. As a result, the islanders became very wealthy. Their per capita income was even higher than that of the United States. They started importing Western foods—sugar, sweets, white bread, meats, and all the delicacies that money could buy. Before long a strange thing happened. Diabetes, obesity, constipation, and other diseases of modern civilization began to appear. According to the World Health Organization up to one-half of the urbanized adult Nauru population have become diabetic.

Protects the Heart

If you want to protect yourself from heart disease, you should include ample amounts of fiber in your diet. A multitude of studies have demonstrated that dietary fiber protects against heart attacks and strokes.[12-14]

Part of the reason why dietary fiber protects the heart is that it reduces many of the risk factors associated with heart disease. Some forms of fiber, such as that found in oat bran, help reduce cholesterol. Blood pressure is also influenced by dietary fiber. Even a modest increase in fiber intake results in a significant decrease in blood pressure.[15, 16] Another risk factor affected by fiber is diabetes. People with diabetes are much more prone to heart disease than the general population. Dietary fiber is known to increase insulin sensitivity, thus reducing symptoms associated with diabetes and, consequently, the risk of heart disease.[17, 18]

If you want to avoid a heart attack or a stroke, you should be eating coconut. Coconut meat is heart healthy. It has a positive impact on blood lipid levels and will *lower* your cholesterol. Studies show that adding coconut into the diet will significantly lower total cholesterol, LDL (bad) cholesterol, triglycerides, and phospholipids. On the other hand, HDL (good) cholesterol increases. So the total lipid profile improves, reducing risk of heart disease. These effects have been observed in both animal and human studies.[19, 20]

Coconut meat not only protects the heart by modifying blood lipid levels, but it also improves antioxidant status and reduces oxidative stress. Antioxidants protect tissues such as the heart and blood vessels from the destructive action of free radicals. Coconut consumption decreases oxidation products in the heart and increases the activity of superoxide dismutase and catalase—antioxidant enzymes that protect the heart and arteries from free radicals that promote atherosclerosis.[21]

Vermifuge

An interesting benefit of coconut fiber, not found in other fibers, is that it acts as a vermifuge (i.e., expels parasitic worms). Eating coconut meat to get rid of parasites is a traditional practice in India that was even recognized among the early medical profession. It was included in a handbook of tropical medicine published in India in 1936[22] and in an Indian Materia Medica with Ayurvedic medicine published in 1976.[23]

In 1984 researchers in India designed a study to test the effectiveness of this traditional remedy.[24] They went to Sadri village in Rajasthan, India where tapeworm infestation was endemic. People here are non-vegetarian and eat raw or improperly cooked beef. Fifty infected individuals volunteered for the study. Various coconut preparations combined with Epsom salt (a strong laxative) were administered to the volunteers. Significant expulsion of parasites occurred when subjects were given either 400 grams of fresh coconut or 200 grams of dried coconut, followed by Epsom salt. The dried coconut was found to be more effective than fresh coconut, and it was determined that after 12 hours, 90 percent of the parasites were expelled. The fresh coconut group expelled only 60 percent of the parasites after 12 hours. Some of the tapeworms that were removed during the study were over six feet long. The health of the patients was monitored afterward for six months. In one third of them no recurrence was found. Among those who had a recurrence the researchers speculated that it was probably caused by reinfestation from eating raw or undercooked meat, a common practice in the area.

At the time of the study the researchers reported that except for Niclosomide, no drug was as effective in the treatment of tapeworm infestation as was coconut. Niclosomide, however, causes tapeworms to waste away or separate, releasing toxins that can cause undesirable side effects. The researchers concluded that since coconut meat is nontoxic, palatable, easily available, and fairly cheap, and because it is highly effective in expelling tapeworms without causing side effects, it is a safe and effective treatment for tapeworm infestation. Since this study verified the effectiveness of this traditional treatment you could honestly say, "a coconut a day flushes the worms away."

Mineral Absorption

The foods with the highest fiber content are seeds and grains like wheat, oats, and flaxseed. One drawback that has been reported by researchers with the bran or fiber from all of these sources is that they contain phytic acid, which binds with minerals in the digestive tract and pulls them out of the body. Consequently, mineral absorption is decreased. Some of the minerals that are bound to phytic acid include zinc, iron, and calcium. It has been suggested that eating too much food containing phytic acid can lead to mineral deficiencies. Even dietary fiber levels of 10 to 20 percent interfere with absorption of minerals in the digestive tract. Yet, we are counseled to get between 20 and 35 percent dietary fiber in our diets. This appears to be a catch-22 situation. We need fiber for good digestive health, but too much may cause nutritional problems. The perfect solution to this problem is not to reduce fiber consumption but to replace some of the fiber we get from grains and seeds with fiber that does not pull minerals out of the body. Coconut fiber fits that description.[25] You can eat all the coconut you want without worrying about it negatively affecting your mineral status.

Types of Fiber

Fiber consists of many components that differ structurally and chemically. There are basically two major classifications of fiber: soluble and insoluble. Each has its own characteristics and benefits.

Soluble fiber partially dissolves in water. It consists of gums, pectins, and mucilages. It is found in abundance in fruits and vegetables. Apple pectin, like that used in making jams and jellies, is a soluble fiber. Its greatest benefit is that it binds onto bile and pulls it out of the body. A major component of bile is cholesterol. By removing bile, less cholesterol is available to be reabsorbed into the body, thus helping to lower total cholesterol levels. Soluble fiber also slows down the digestion and assimilation of sugars, thus moderating blood sugar levels.

Insoluble fiber cannot be dissolved in water. It consists of lignin, cellulose, and hemicellulose, which are the structural or woody portions of plants. It is found primarily in grains, nuts, and legumes. Wheat bran is mostly an insoluble fiber. This is the type of fiber we usually think of as roughage. It softens stools and regulates intestinal transit time.

There are significant differences in the effects of these two types of fiber. Evidence shows that dietary fiber from both soluble and insoluble sources is essential for health. Most plant foods contain a mixture of both. Because insoluble fiber has a much greater influence on intestinal transit time, it is considered the more significant in terms of health benefits. Complications that arise from a sluggish bowel set up the conditions that lead to most of the health problems caused by a lack of dietary fiber. Many studies have shown the superiority of wheat bran, which is high in insoluble fiber, over the fiber in fruits and vegetables, which are composed primarily of soluble fiber. Insoluble fiber is primarily responsible for providing protection from cancer, heart disease, diabetes, Crohn's disease, and other intestinal problems.[26-29] Wheat bran, because of its high concentration of insoluble fiber, has been repeatedly recommended for these conditions.

Like wheat bran, coconut is composed primarily of insoluble fiber. The fiber in coconut is about 93 percent insoluble and 7 percent soluble. Despite the low percentage of soluble fiber, coconut still contains a significant amount of this fiber. In fact, it contains more soluble fiber than either wheat or rice. So it has just as much effect in reducing cholesterol and modulating blood sugar levels as most other high-fiber plant foods, perhaps even more because insoluble fiber also affects these conditions to some extent. Its real advantage is that it contains a higher percentage of insoluble fiber than wheat bran, thus making it potentially more effective in protecting against digestive health problems.

Coconut Flour and Dietary Fiber

You can get the benefits of coconut fiber by eating fresh or dried coconut and adding coconut to recipes. Most people are familiar with seeing coconut used in cookies, cakes, and pies and get the mistaken impression that coconut is used only for desserts and candies. You don't have to eat sweets to get the benefit of coconut fiber. Another way to increase your fiber consumption is though coconut flour.

Coconut flour is made from coconut meat. It is dried, defatted, and finely ground into a powder resembling wheat flour. Like other flours, it can be used in making bread, muffins, cookies, and casseroles. The only drawback is that it does not contain gluten—the protein found in many grains. Gluten is important in baked goods because it makes dough sticky, allowing it to trap and hold air bubbles, which makes bread light and fluffy. Breads made from flours that lack gluten are often dense and hard. However, if you are allergic to gluten, as many people are, not having this may be a benefit.

With coconut flour, you can make a wide variety of baked goods that are low in digestible carbohydrate and high in fiber. Coconut flour has a much higher fiber and a lower digestible carbohydrate content than other flours. It contains about four times as much fiber as soy flour. Although it doesn't contain gluten, it does not lack protein. It has more protein than enriched white flour, rye flour, or cornmeal and has about the same as buckwheat and whole wheat flours.

In most cases coconut flour cannot be substituted completely for wheat or other flours in standard bread recipes. You need to combine it with wheat, rye, or oat flour. When making quick breads, you can generally replace up to 25 percent of the wheat flour with coconut flour. This still increases the fiber content considerably.

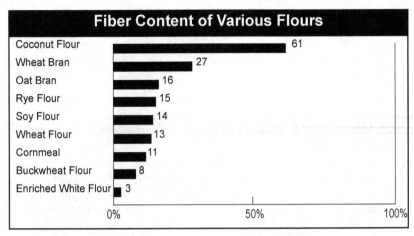

Fiber Content of Various Flours

Flour	Percentage
Coconut Flour	61
Wheat Bran	27
Oat Bran	16
Rye Flour	15
Soy Flour	14
Wheat Flour	13
Cornmeal	11
Buckwheat Flour	8
Enriched White Flour	3

Coconut flour contains the highest percentage of dietary fiber in comparison to other flours. Sixty-one percent of the flour consists of fiber with water, protein, fat, and carbohydrate making up the remaining 39 percent.

You cannot use standard bread recipes using 100 percent coconut flour. The characteristics of the flour are significantly different from wheat. However, with the right approach you can make delicious breads, muffins, cakes, cookies, and a variety of other flour-based products using only coconut flour. The results are every bit as good, and in many cases even better, than wheat flour. For people who are allergic to wheat, coconut flour makes an ideal replacement. For recipes using 100 percent coconut flour I recommend my book *Cooking with Coconut Flour: A Delicious Low-Carb, Gluten-Free Alternative to Wheat.*

Coconut flour can also be used like a dietary fiber supplement. You use only a tablespoon or so and add it to beverages, smoothies, baked goods, casseroles, soups, and hot cereal. This makes a simple and easy way to add fiber into your daily diet without making drastic changes in the way you eat.

Research shows that adding even a little fiber to the diet can have a significant influence on health. For example, in a study on cardiovascular disease, a high-fiber diet was associated with a 21 percent lower risk of heart disease. The difference in fiber intake of the subjects wasn't great. The highest intake was only 23 grams, only about 8 or 9 grams above average. Eight or nine grams of fiber can easily be added to the diet by substituting whole wheat bread for white, eating whole grain cereal, or adding a little more high-fiber foods, such as coconut. Nutritionists tell us that we should get between 20 and 35 grams of fiber a day. Dr. Burkitt recommends 40 grams a day. Eating 35 to 40 grams of fiber a day would be ideal; however, increasing your fiber intake by even a small amount can have beneficial effects. Adding as little as 2 or 3 tablespoons of coconut fiber a day to your diet may be all you need to take advantage of many of the health benefits coconut has to offer.

COCONUT WATER
The Fluid of Life

"Coconut water is sweet, increasing semen, promoting digestion, and clearing the urinary path," says Ayurvedic medicine of India. Coconut water, also called coconut juice, is the liquid found inside a fresh coconut. Contrary to popular belief, this liquid is *not* the same as coconut milk. Coconut milk is entirely different and is discussed more fully in the next section.

Coconut water is a relatively clear liquid that looks more like water than it does milk. It is very sweet and tasty and is a favorite beverage among Asian and Pacific Islanders. In addition to natural sugars, it contains a complex array of vitamins and minerals, which makes it a nutritious beverage. It is high in potassium, chlorides, calcium, and magnesium, with a modest amount of sodium, sugar, and protein. It is essentially fat-free. While the mineral content remains fairly constant, the sugar and protein concentrations increase as the nut matures.

Coconut water contains a variety of nutrients including trace minerals which come directly from the sea and which most other foods lack. Coconut palms grow abundantly throughout most of the tropics. Even the tiniest islands are covered with palms littering the ground with fallen nuts. All that is needed to quench one's thirst is to reach for the nearest coconut. On many small islands, coconut water is the only potable water available. For these reasons coconut water has been a lifesaver for many people and has been referred to as the "fluid of life."

The electrolyte profile of coconut water is somewhat similar to human plasma and for that reason it has been used by doctors as an intravenous solution and injected directly into the bloodstream to prevent dehydration. When freshly extracted from the coconut, this liquid is free from germs and parasites. Doctors working in tropical climates have often used the water from coconuts as IV solutions, a common practice during World War II and in Vietnam where commercial IV solutions were often in short supply.[30] Water from an unopened coconut is uncontaminated by bacteria, fungi, or other pathogens. Therefore, if prepared properly, it can be given intravenously without fear of introducing harmful microorganisms. Recent research on the use of coconut water as an intravenous fluid has shown it to compare favorably with commercial solutions.[31] Coconut water does not harm red blood cells, is non-allergenic, and is readily accepted by the body. It is considered a safe and useful means of rehydration, particularly when a patient suffers from a potassium deficiency.[32] In fact, coconut water has been shown to be just as effective as commercial electrolyte solutions in prolonging survival time in sick patients.[33] Researchers have demonstrated that coconut water can be given through intravenous infusion by as much as one fourth to one third of the patient's body weight without complications.

Coconut water is also highly recommended as a means for oral rehydration.[34] The water has been useful in tropical areas to overcome diarrheal dehydration. Diarrhea is a major health problem in many underdeveloped countries killing nearly five million children each year. Excessive physical activity can also cause dehydration. Athletes and sports enthusiasts use coconut water to replenish electrolytes lost in perspiration. It works just as well and even better than some popular commercial sports drinks. Coconut water is a natural sports drink.

The taste of coconut water varies depending on the age of the coconut. The water from green (immature) coconuts is regarded as the best in taste and quality. The water from mature coconuts, although good, doesn't compare. Unfortunately, unless you live where coconuts are grown, it is difficult to get green coconuts. Until recently, just about the only way to get coconut water was to crack open a coconut. The demand for a natural sports drink has led to the commercial packaging of young coconut water. It is now available in many locations in bottled and Tetra Pak containers.

Cholesterol Control

Coconut water is more than just a sports drink or nutritious beverage. It is a health tonic. Research has shown that it has a positive effect on cholesterol. In one study, for example, blood cholesterol levels of HDL—the good cholesterol that protects against heart disease—increased by 46.2 percent.[35] The researchers indicated that liver cholesterol levels were reduced by 26.3 percent and risk of atherosclerosis (hardening of the arteries) decreased by 41.1 percent. Their conclusion was that coconut water is a natural, nutritious drink that could help prevent the formation of atherosclerosis and protect against heart disease.

Urinary and Reproductive Systems

Coconut water has long been known for its therapeutic effect on the urinary and reproductive systems. It is reported to clear bladder infections, remove kidney stones, and improve sexual vitality. Medical research has shown consumption of coconut water to be very effective in dissolving kidney stones.[36] Dr. Eugenio Macalalag, director of the urology department at the Chinese

General Hospital in the Philippines, says that coconut water has demonstrated its effectiveness in patients suffering from kidney and urethral stone problems. His patients have even been able to suspend dialysis treatment after regular oral intake of coconut water. In the Philippines coconut water is commonly known as buko juice. Dr. Macalalag has also reported success in patients by directly infusing the water into the kidneys. He calls the treatment bukolysis. A saying that has now become popular in the Philippines is: "A coconut a day keeps the urologist away."

Coconut water injected through urethral catheters inserted up to where the stones are lodged (bukolysis) has resulted in significant daily decrease in size, disintegration of the stones, and expulsion without the need for surgery. Even by oral intake coconut water, taken 2 or 3 times a week, has been observed to result in significant size reduction of kidney stones within a short time. Macalalag reports that, of his 1,670 patients who were recurrent stone formers and who took buko therapy, only 13 percent had recurrence of stones in a 10-year period, and the stones were small and passed out easily. Coconut water therapy is so effective that kidney stone patients are spared going through expensive medical procedures. Dr. Macalalag jokingly complains that because of this he has suffered from "AIDS" or what he calls "acute income deficiency syndrome."

Coconut water is a natural diuretic so it increases urine flow. This helps to dilute the urine so that stones are less likely to form and helps to flush existing stones out. It also is helpful in preventing bladder infections.

Not only does coconut water clean out the urinary tract, it revitalizes the reproductive system. Coconut water from fresh green coconuts is reputed to increase libido and enhance performance. No need for Viagra here; coconut water will keep you young and virile. It doesn't work only for men; women in their mid-60s have reported an increase in libido after drinking young coconut water. Water from a *mature* coconut, however, doesn't seem to have as strong an effect. It must be from a fresh immature or green coconut.

Glaucoma

Coconut water could be useful for those who have glaucoma. Glaucoma occurs when fluid pressure in the eye becomes abnormally high, causing damage to tiny blood vessels and optic nerve fibers. If left untreated, glaucoma can lead to permanent loss of vision. There is no cure for glaucoma; all that can be done is to prevent it from worsening. Treatment consists of putting medication in the eye to relieve pressure. Medicated eye drops must be used on a regular basis to keep the fluid pressure under control. Coconut water has proven to be effective in significantly reducing fluid pressure in the eyes.[37] The water is not put in the eyes but taken orally. The effect lasts for 2½ hours.

PROPERTIES OF COCONUT WATER

In India coconut water is considered a nutritious wholesome beverage with many medicinal properties among which are the following:

- Reduces problems for infants suffering from intestinal disturbances.
- Is an effective oral rehydration medium.
- Contains organic compounds possessing growth-promoting properties.
- Keeps the body cool.
- Used topically it prevents prickly heat and summer boils and relieves rashes caused by smallpox, chicken pox, measles, etc.
- Kills intestinal worms.
- Presence of saline and albumen makes it a good drink in cholera cases.
- Checks urinary infections.
- Excellent tonic for the old and sick.
- Cures malnourishment.
- Diuretic.
- Dissolves kidney and urethral stones.
- Useful as an intravenous solution.
- Useful as blood plasma substitute and is readily accepted by the body.
- Aids the quick absorption of drugs and makes their peak concentration in the blood easier by its electrolytic effect.
- Urinary antiseptic and eliminates poisons in case of mineral poisoning.

Source: Coconut Development Board, India.

In addition, coconut water has shown to act as an antioxidant, scavenging many types of destructive free radicals and protecting hemoglobin in the blood from nitrite-induced oxidation.[38] These effects are most significant when using fresh coconut water. They diminish significantly when the water is heated or processed.

A traditional method for treating cataract involves the use of coconut water. Several drops of coconut water are put into the eyes, a hot damp washcloth is placed over the eyes, the patient then lies down with the washcloth in place for about 10 minutes. I know of people getting good results with this procedure. Perhaps part of the reason it may work is due to the antioxidant effect of coconut water. Cataracts are caused by oxidation so the antioxidant effect of the water might be of some help.

Laxative

One thing to be aware of when using coconut water is that drinking too much can have a laxative effect. This characteristic of coconut water may or may not be desirable depending on the normal frequency of bowel movements. For those who are constipated, drinking lots of coconut water may be a good thing. For everyone else, consumption may be best limited to bowel tolerance. Bowel tolerance is the maximum amount of coconut water you can drink without experiencing loose stools. Most people can drink a couple of glassed of coconut water without problem. This will vary with each individual. Bowel tolerance may increase with regular use.

The many health benefits of coconut water, including its anti-cancer and anti-aging properties, are described in more detail in my book *Coconut Water for Health and Healing.*

COCONUT MILK

Coconut milk is not the watery liquid you find sloshing around inside a fresh coconut. It is a product obtained by extracting the juice out of coconut meat. Its taste, appearance, and nutrient content are very different from coconut water.

Coconut water has almost no fat or protein. Coconut milk is rich in fat and protein. It has a thick creamy texture and is solid white in color, giving it an appearance similar to cow's milk. Coconut milk contains about 17 to 24 percent fat, depending on how much water is used in processing. The higher fat milk is often called coconut cream and is very thick and rich, just like dairy cream.

Another difference between coconut water and milk is the sugar content. Coconut water is sweet. Coconut milk is not. Although coconut milk has a pleasant taste, it contains little sugar. It even has less sugar than dairy milk. Because of its low carbohydrate content, coconut milk is ideal for low-carb diets. Coconut milk is very popular in Asian cooking particularly in Thailand and the Philippines. In some communities it is used in preparing virtually every meal.

A variety of prepared coconut milk products are available commercially. They are usually sold in 14-ounce cans but are also available in larger cans as well as in cartons. Coconut milk usually contains about 17 percent fat. Coconut cream contains about 21 to 24 percent fat. Some coconut milk is watered down to reduce the fat content. This is called "low-fat" or "light" coconut milk. The fat content is 14 percent or less. To retain the milk's thick texture, thickeners such as guar gum are sometimes added. I usually avoid low-fat milks because the coconut oil content is reduced. One of the reasons I eat coconut milk is to get the benefit of the fat. I don't want to reduce the benefit by eating low-fat

Libido

I went to the little Vietnamese grocery store earlier today to buy a whole case of coconut milk. The little old lady shopkeeper held up her hand like a traffic cop, but she had an impish smile on her face.

She asked me, "You buy lotsa coconut milk with good fat! Not watery stuff. You want live 100 year?"

I nodded my head affirmatively and smiled at her.

She warned me with mock sternness in her voice "All this coconut milk! You clothes no fit soon. You get skinny and have to buy new clothes."

I said I could live with that.

She then said. "You get like young man and get girl in trouble like years ago."

This one took me by surprise. I had not heard of this property of coconuts. I smiled and said I could live with that also.

She smiled at me and said, "I bet you could!" Giggled at me and blushed.

As I was leaving the store, the woman said "I from Thailand. We know these things about coconut. You be back soon. One case not last you long."

I never heard about high fat coconut milk or coconut oil being good for restoring libido in older men.

Alobar

---

milk. In my opinion, the higher the fat content, the better. Another product you may run across is *cream of coconut*. This is not the same as coconut cream. Cream of coconut is coconut cream with added sugar and is very sweet. It is used in making sweet beverages and desserts.

A Good Source of Coconut Oil

Because coconut milk contains a high percentage of fat, the health benefits are the same as those of coconut oil. It can be used topically in many cases like the oil. For instance, it can be and is applied on the skin to treat cuts, burns, and sunburn. It is good for the scalp and hair. It can help control dandruff and makes hair shiny and healthy looking. It can help keep the skin soft and silky smooth and is reported to be a good wrinkle remover. Fermented coconut milk is used to get rid of head lice. Internally it is said to be good for sore throat as well as relieving stomach ulcers. In fact, any condition that is affected by coconut oil will be similarly affected by coconut milk.

The primary advantages coconut milk has over pure coconut oil is that it is easier to extract from the meat and is more versatile and can be used in far more ways in food preparation. Coconut milk provides an easy way to add coconut oil into the diet. Coconut milk makes an excellent substitute for dairy. It has a rich, creamy texture and mild coconut flavor. It can be used in just about any way you would use dairy milk and cream. Like dairy milk, it is not sweet so it can be used to make a variety of savory dishes such as soups, chowders, stews, curries, and sauces and, of course, it can be used in making desserts as well. It is a good substitute for milk and can be consumed by the glass or used to make beverages and smoothies.

A Dairy-Free Milk

For people who can't or don't want to use dairy, coconut milk is a healthy alternative. Many people are lactose intolerant or allergic to dairy. Some don't eat dairy because they are vegetarian or prefer not to consume milk that has been pasteurized, homogenized, fractionated, or otherwise manipulated by modern food processing. Some people who prefer raw foods don't drink milk or other dairy products because it has been heated during processing. Regardless of the reason, these people can eat coconut milk and still enjoy the "taste" of dairy products.

Allergies are a major problem with many people. Over 60 percent of all food allergies are to milk and nuts.[39] The good news for these people is that they have an alternative with coconut. While people can be allergic to most any type of food, relatively few people have allergic reactions to coconut. Based on medical research and clinical observation, coconut is considered a hypoallergenic food and, therefore, is recommend as a nutritious substitute in the diet for those who are troubled by allergies.[40] Forty-three percent of all those who have food allergies are allergic to tree nuts—walnuts, pecans, almonds, etc. People who are allergic to nuts, however, are not generally allergic to coconut. Although it is possible to be allergic to coconuts, coconut allergy in people with tree nut allergy is extremely rare. In fact, only two cases in the entire world have ever been reported.[41] So people with food allergies, particularly nut allergies, can eat coconut and coconut milk without fear.

Eating coconut may actually help relieve symptoms associated with some allergies. Many people have reported improvement in allergy symptoms when they use coconut regularly in their diets. Part of the reason is that coconut oil helps balance the environment in the intestines and heals the intestinal wall— two things that can significantly influence the occurrence of allergies.

Coconut Culture

Throughout history people from all over the world have developed methods of preserving foods by fermentation. Raw milk from cows, sheep, goats, yaks, and camels is preserved by culturing it with bacteria. These harmless bacteria are effective in suppressing spoilage and disease-causing organisms, making it possible to preserve milk for several days or weeks without refrigeration. Cultured products have become ethnic favorites and have been introduced around the world as people have migrated from place to place. Yogurt is perhaps the most commonly recognized cultured milk. It is believed to have originated with nomadic tribes of Eastern Europe and Western Asia and has been a staple in Middle Eastern diets for centuries. The word "yogurt" is of Turkish origin.

There are many different types of fermented milks. They all differ in taste and texture from one another by the type of organisms used in the fermentation process. Originally the bacteria in milk appeared naturally and contained dozens of different organisms. Kefir, for instance, contains nearly 50 separate organisms. Because the types of organisms carried through the air varies from region to region and from season to season, milk, even that from the same locality, can vary in taste and quality. At times it may be better than at others. It was almost impossible to get the exact same results each time, relying strictly on nature. When a good quality culture was obtained, it was preserved by starting a new batch using a portion from the previous one. In this way the best cultures were preserved.

Each region developed their own unique cultured products, for instance, kefir from the Caucasian mountains of Southern Russia, fil mjolk from Scandinavia, and nata de coco from the Philippines.

Cultured milk gained a reputation as a health food that could help individuals retain youthfulness and restore health and vitality to the sick. Modern interest in cultured milk began in 1920 when Russian researcher Ilya Metchnikoff reported that Bulgarian peasants, whose diet included a great deal of yogurt, were unusually healthy and lived to extraordinary ages.

Metchnikoff believed that the secret to the health benefits of cultured milk came from the organisms involved in the fermentation process. These "friendly" bacteria are much the same as those that inhabit our intestinal tract. Each of us has billions of microorganisms (bacteria and yeasts) in our digestive tract. These organisms are essential for good health as they aid in digestion, enhance nutrient absorption, support the immune system, inhibit the growth of disease-causing organisms, and protect us from infections.

Two of the most common bacteria found in cultured milk as well as in our digestive tract are Lactobacillus and Bifidobacteria. These friendly bacteria act as sentinels, constantly on guard protecting us from harmful organisms. The ability of these friendly bacteria to ward off attacks from disease-causing organisms is incredible. They actively block harmful bacteria and yeast from attacking and harming cells within the intestinal tract. Not only do they protect our cells from harm, but they also prohibit the growth of harmful organisms.

Lactobacillus, for example, prevents the growth of *Staphylococcus aureus*, a pathogenic organism that causes food poising, urinary tract infections, and toxic shock syndrome among other problems. Researchers have shown that wounds infected with staphylococcus heal quicker when Lactobacillus is present.[42] They found that while the germs were not killed by the Lactobacillus, they stopped multiplying, allowing the body's defenses to fight off the infection.

According to a study in *The Lancet*, the British Medical Association Journal, treating pregnant women with "good bacteria" such as Lactobacillus in yogurt may prevent their future children from developing asthma.

Friendly microorganisms in fermented milk produce compounds that inhibit the activity of enzymes involved in the formation of cancer within the intestinal tract and protect against colon and rectal cancers. But the benefits don't stop there. The influence bacteria have goes beyond the intestinal tract. The anti-cancer substances produced by friendly bacteria also reduce risk of cancers elsewhere in the body. Several studies have shown a reduced risk of breast cancer in women who consume fermented milk products.[43-45]

Along with the friendly bacteria in our digestive tract, we also have not-so-friendly bacteria and yeasts—organisms that promote disease. The only thing that keeps them from causing illness is the good bacteria. If the good bacteria were not there, the bad bacteria and yeasts would take over and wreak havoc on our health. Unfortunately, this happens all too often. Drugs often affect the microflora in the intestine. Antibiotics can't tell the difference between the good and the bad bacteria. A single course of antibiotics meant to kill an infection will knock out friendly gut bacteria as well. Without the protection of good bacteria, yeasts such as candida, which are not affected by antibiotics, proliferate and lead to yeast infections and candidiasis.

Foods also affect intestinal health. The environment in the intestines is like an ecosystem in nature. If one element of the ecosystem is unbalanced, everything else is affected. The food we eat sets the stage for the environment in the intestines. A diet rich in refined carbohydrates and sweets feeds yeast cells and encourages their growth. Dietary fiber feeds friendly bacteria. A diet that is low in fiber and high in processed flour and sugar disrupts the natural environment, causing an imbalance in the microflora of the gut. Consequently, the acid-alkaline balance shifts, favoring the growth of unhealthy organisms and further inhibiting the growth of protective bacteria. Without the full protection of the good bacteria, the immune system becomes stressed and health suffers.

A number of health problems can arise when intestinal health is out of balance. Good bacteria produce many of the vitamins we need for optimal health such as vitamins B-6, B-12, K, niacin, and folic acid. If intestinal health is poor, production of these vitamins is reduced. If you eat a well-balanced diet it isn't too much of a problem but if your diet is poor, then you are already lacking these important nutrients and a reduction can promote nutritional deficiencies.

Friendly bacteria also help suppress activity that converts harmless chemicals into carcinogenic agents. So intestinal health influences your susceptibly to cancer. A host of health problems can arise from having poor intestinal health, including constipation, irritable bowel syndrome, hemorrhoids, allergies, hay fever, colds, chronic fatigue, migraines, ulcers, etc. To put it simply: if your gut ain't happy, you ain't happy.

Coconut can be an aid in normalizing the environment and improving the function of the digestive tract. The high-fiber content of coconut meat helps eliminate constipation and keep things moving along properly. The fiber is also used as food by friendly bacteria, encouraging their growth. The medium-chain fatty acids in coconut oil kill candida and disease-causing bacteria that compete for space in the digestive tract with friendly bacteria. MCFA do not harm friendly bacteria. Cultured coconut milk and water provide reinforcements that increase the number of good bacteria in the gut.

Nata de coco is a fermented product indigenous to the Philippines made from coconut water and sometimes the milk. Coconut farmers make it at home and eat it as a dessert. Like yogurt and other cultured milks, sugar and fruit are often added. Nata de coco, however, is very different from yogurt. It has a mild flavor, a translucent gelatin-like appearance, and a chewy texture. Unlike cultured dairy, it is a good source of dietary fiber. The fiber is from bacterial cellulose, which gives it its distinctive chewy texture. It is considered a health food in the Philippines because it is a rich source of fiber and low in calories. Since it has near zero calories, it makes an ideal bulk diet food. It can help fill you up without filling you out. It is also reported to prevent gastrointestinal disorders and even colon cancer, and has even been used as a dressing for wounds. Although it originated in the Philippines, it has become immensely popular in Japan and other Asian countries.

In recent years a new cultured coconut product has emerged that combines the legendary health benefits of kefir from the Caucasian Mountains with the wonders of coconut from the tropics. This new cultured sensation is kefir coconut milk and coconut water.

Chapter 7

HOW TO BE HAPPY, HEALTHY, AND BEAUTIFUL

In this chapter I explain how to use coconut to improve your heath and prevent illness. You will learn how to use it externally as well as internally. As Paul Sorse claimed, it will make you "happy, healthy, and beautiful." The experience of Popi Laudico given below describes how coconut oil can change lives. She truly feels happy, healthy, and beautiful.

"I have always believed that if you open your mind and your heart to the possibility of wonderful things happening to you, the universe will seek them out and make sure they come your way. One such life changing event happened to me when one of my Tai Chi classmates asked me if I wanted to try a new product that their company was developing. I had been buying essential patchouli oil from her and she wanted to know if I was interested in virgin coconut oil. 'What does it do?' I inquired and she said it was very good for the skin among other things and that all I had to do was put it all over and drink it.

"I have always been plagued by various skin conditions brought about by allergic reactions to a great number of stimulations from dust to almost everything I ate. My reactions would all come out on my skin. It was so bad that my friends—out of pity—would give me the numbers of their dermatologists so I could get help. At that point my bathroom already resembled a small apothecary so I was willing to try anything.

"I must say that from the first time I oiled myself from head to foot it was immediate love. I guess I must have known, even if I had not consciously known it then, that the light yummy smelling oil would save me. After a month of religiously using it, the compliments started pouring in and they haven't stopped until this day—three years later.

"Now when I visit a dermatologist to get a facial, they marvel at how under a magnifying lens my skin resembles that of a baby. Now that kind of compliment was something I was completely unaccustomed to. And instead of selling me their services, they insist I do not leave without giving them my source for the oil. Even doctors who have treated my numerous skin conditions marvel at how truly healthy my skin looks. And that's the key to this whole miracle—health.

"The oil managed to cleanse me in and out and has improved my resistance to the things I was previously so allergic to. I have not taken my allergy medicines nor have I taken any shots since I've been drinking the oil. And the glow on my skin comes from within. I have a lifestyle that keeps me under the sun more often than not—a big no-no when it comes to most cosmetic treatments, but not for this oil. Now all the sun does is kiss my cheeks and give it a nice rosy glow. Amazing.

"And I do not have any visible scars from my war torn dermal past. Friends who've never seen me before do not believe the stories of scars over scars over scars, while old friends vouch that it's been such a transformation. I'm practically a walking-talking billboard for what this simple yet wonderful gift from nature can do, and continues to do.

"Since that first drink I've learned more about this virgin coconut oil and a lot of publicity has come out about it. It really should be a part of everyone's daily routine. When I realized what it was and all that it can do, I will never be without it. And I will continue to tell those who care to listen about how it has changed my life and made me more beautiful and healthier."

USING COCONUT EXTERNALLY

Every year I plant a garden in my back yard. One summer I spent several hours working under the hot sun. I could feel the skin on my arms and neck beginning to burn. I knew I should do something, but I was so involved that I stayed out several more hours. When I finally did come in, my exposed skin was as red as a beet and very painful. When I took my shower, the warm water burned my sensitive skin. I knew I would be hurting for the next day or two, and my skin would peel terribly just as it had many times in the past.

After my shower it hurt so bad that I grabbed some coconut oil hoping it might help moisturize the skin and soothe the pain. Within a half hour all the pain had vanished and the redness had faded. I couldn't believe it. I didn't expect the oil to do this; I used it just to keep the skin from drying out and from getting worse. I was elated. I had found something that could heal sunburned skin.

If it could heal my sunburn, I wondered, what would happen if I put it on *before* I went out into the sun? The next week I put a layer of oil on all my exposed skin and went out in the yard. I spent at least 6 hours under the hot sun. Normally this long would have burnt me to a crisp. But I had no sunburn pain at all. Instead of turning red, as I normally would, my skin developed a very light tan. I was thrilled. The only place I got sunburned was on the top of my head where my hair is very thin. I didn't put any oil on my scalp because I wore a hat and didn't think I needed it there. But my hat had several tiny holes in it and the sun penetrated through these holes and burnt the top of my head. A few days later the skin on my head peeled just as it always does when I get sunburned. The skin on my neck and arms that was exposed to the full intensity of the sun never hurt and did not peel. I became an instant believer in the healing power of coconut oil.

I learned the reason why islanders apply coconut oil to their skin every morning. Traditionally, they wear next to nothing and live in an environment where they are under the hot burning tropical sun every day. The oil protects them from the burning rays of the sun. Consequently, they have smooth, beautiful skin, and *no* skin cancer. They live under the intense tropical sun, yet skin cancer is rare.

The traditional remedy among islanders for burns as well as cuts, bruises, sprains, insect bites, and other injuries is to apply coconut oil to the injured area. It not only heals injuries but skin problems of almost every kind. It cleanses the skin from acne, soothes rashes, and kills skin and nail fungus such as athlete's foot, jock itch, and ringworm. Even age spots and wrinkles show improvement when massaged daily with coconut oil.

I don't think there is a skin condition that coconut oil can't help. I was in my yard one afternoon cleaning up some old wood and trash. In the process I uncovered a large number of spider nests. At the end of the day I noticed several spider bites on my arm. The bites were very itchy and swollen. I massaged coconut oil into my arm and within a short time the itching stopped and the swelling subsided. I thought no more of the matter. Two days later I discovered that a spot on my back, which had an annoying itch, was also covered in spider bites. I noticed that the bites on my back were swollen and inflamed while the ones on my arm, which were treated with coconut oil, were barely noticeable. I rubbed in the oil and the itchy area and inflammation soon faded away. Coconut oil never ceases to amaze me.

Some people hesitate to eat the oil because they've been told it's bad for them. I explain that they don't need to consume the oil to experience the benefits. All they need to do is put it on their skin. That's it. Most are willing to do this. Once you start applying the oil to the skin on a regular basis, you will see a transformation. Rough, dry, flaky skin starts to become smooth, soft, and younger looking. Acne, psoriasis, and other skin problems begin to disappear. The skin looks and feels healthier because it is healthier. Whenever I meet someone who has doubts about the healing powers of coconut oil, I tell

Dermatitis and Acne

When I take my morning dose, I've been rubbing some on my hands that have eczema and after a few days of this, it's disappearing! No more flaking, itching or blisters!

Cathy

My sister has had a horrible, painful rash on her lower legs for some time now. They have injected her calves with steroid shots, steroid creams and more, with little to almost no improvement. On a recent family vacation with her, I rubbed coconut oil on her legs and the very next DAY she saw amazing improvement. Her skin was all smooth, and though still somewhat discolored, of course, it was already improving the color of her skin as well. She was amazed. I wasn't. I knew it would work.

Sharon

My grandson (17 years old) has used prescribed meds for 3 or 4 years now for acne…The meds haven't worked for him. About 6 weeks ago I gave him some virgin coconut oil to use on his face…His acne has cleared up just fine. He uses regular soap to wash. Now his sister is starting to develop acne also and she came to me and asked for some of the good stuff that I gave to her brother.

James

I started using the oil on my skin and hair and I'm amazed by the quick results. My hair is much softer/shinier even after one day. Also my son put some on last night before bed. He told me this morning that he usually wakes up with a few little whitehead pimples on his chin and this morning his face was clearer. He is very excited about it.

Gail

them not to take my word for it, but try it themselves. That's all they have to do to become believers. What it does to the outside of the body it will do on the inside—make you look and feel younger and healthier.

Daily Skin Care

Pacific Islanders have a tradition of applying coconut oil to their skin from head to toe every morning. They have learned that it protects them from the blistering rays of the hot tropical sun and keeps their skin smooth and healthy. Using coconut oil as a daily skin lotion will strengthen the skin and underlying tissues, help protect it from injury, promote and speed healing, and fend off invading germs that cause infection and illness. Your skin will look and feel softer and healthier.

One of the primary functions of the skin is to act as a barrier to disease-causing germs and parasites. It is more than just a physical barrier but a chemical one as well. Oil and sweat secreted by the body produce a chemical environment that is inhospitable to most disease-causing germs. Harmful germs find it difficult to live in this environment so their numbers are relatively low. The skin is slightly acidic, about 5.0 on the pH scale.

The body's natural oil, sebum, contains medium-chain triglycerides similar to those in coconut oil. On the surface of our skin live lipophilic bacteria. These bacteria are important to our health. They consume the glycerol portion of the oil on our skin, leaving the fatty acids. In this process they convert medium-chain triglycerides (MCTs) in the sebum into potent antimicrobial MCFAs that kill harmful bacteria, viruses, and fungi. Our entire body is covered by a thin protective layer of MCFAs produced by this bacteria. Medium-chain fatty *acids*, as the name implies, are acidic, thus they also help to establish the body's protective acid layer.

MCTs in coconut oil or sebum or any other source do not exhibit any antimicrobial properties. This is important to understand. Only when MCTs are digested and converted into MCFAs are the germ fighting characteristics activated. This is why fresh coconut can spoil and go moldy. Coconut oil applied on the skin, therefore, does not kill bacteria immediately. In order to activate its antimicrobial power it must first be converted into MCFAs by digestive enzymes or skin bacteria.

Ironically, every time you bathe with soap and water, you wash off the skin's natural protective layer. After a bath when you feel you are the cleanest, you are actually most vulnerable to infection. The protective acid layer and MCFAs have been removed. Applying a thin layer of coconut oil will help to quickly reestablish your body's natural chemical barrier.

For full protection the oil should be applied over the entire body from the soles of the feet to the top of the head. You don't need to use much. A teaspoon or so is plenty for the entire body. Wherever the skin is thick, rough, scaly, dry, bumpy, damaged, discolored or otherwise affected, massage the oil into the skin and allow it to soak in. The oil should be rubbed or massaged into the skin and not simply brushed on like a layer of paint. You should work it into the skin for best results. Don't use too much oil. The skin will absorb the oil to the point of saturation. After which, the oil will simply pool on the surface of the skin and just be wiped off on your clothes. Apply just enough that it will soak completely into the skin in about 10 minutes. If needed, you can reapply the oil after an hour or so.

Don't be afraid of putting the oil on your face. If you don't use too much, it will not make your face look greasy. It will actually improve your complexion and appearance. Excessively dry skin may need several applications. Coconut oil isn't like many commercial creams that leave a greasy film. Some people with very dry skin like this film because it keeps the skin from drying out. These creams and lotions don't do anything to heal the skin; they're only a temporary fix that must be repeated for life and, despite their use, skin conditions generally get worse with age. Coconut oil, on the other hand, works to heal the skin. In time the skin will improve.

Coconut oil gives the skin a youthful shiny appearance, which is especially noticeable on the face. It is an excellent natural exfoliant that can help shed ugly dead skin cells. When the skin is unable to exfoliate naturally, the surface of the skin begins to build up old cells. The appearance of the skin becomes dull and, in severe cases, flaky. Coconut oil encourages the shedding of excess layers of dead cells revealing smooth skin and a youthful, healthy complexion.

Massage Oil

Coconut oil makes the best massage oil because of its healing properties. It improves skin health and appearance and helps soothe tight and sore muscles. It's also considered a non-staining oil. This is important to massage therapists who use sheets in their work. Unlike other oils, it is less likely to stain and ruin them. However, if you use too much coconut oil and soak it into the sheet, it will leave a stain, but not as bad as other oils do.

Pure coconut oil is an excellent massage oil. Coconut oil, however, absorbs quickly, so many massage therapists combine a good quality monounsaturated oil, such as almond oil at a ratio of 1 part almond oil and 2 parts coconut oil. This gives the oil more lubrication so that the hands can glide easily over the skin.

Oils are readily absorbed into the skin and bloodstream of both the client and massage therapist. Care should be used in choosing oils that are healthy. A rule of thumb: if you wouldn't eat it then don't use it on the skin.

Massage

A few months ago, I switched over to coconut oil in my massage work using it for a full body massage. Most notable are the results from the women I've used this on. Their skin has a nice tone and color to it now and they remark how so much better their skin feels and looks. Using it on a lady, all her little bumps and small scabs disappeared on her upper back leaving her skin very smooth and pleasant to the touch.
Tracy

Hair Care

Coconut oil can do wonders for your hair. It will give it a shine and healthy luster as well as enrich its natural color. Some claim that it helps prevent both premature graying and baldness. It is also great for the scalp and helps control dandruff.

As a hair treatment, apply a liberal amount of oil to your scalp and work it in. One to two teaspoons of oil is a good amount. Work it in like a massage. The hair and scalp should be completely coated in oil but not so much as to be dripping wet. Allow the oil time to soak in. The longer you can wait before washing it out the better. I recommend at least 15 minutes and preferably 30 to 60 minutes, longer if possible. You may want to do this the first thing in the morning upon arising and keep it on as long as you can before showering. Another option is to apply the oil at night before going to bed. Put on a shower cap, sleep with it on, and wash your hair out in the morning. You will be amazed at how bright and shiny your hair looks and how well coconut oil controls dandruff.

Coconut milk is also known as an excellent hair conditioner, giving hair body and luster. Use it as you would the oil. It is reported that using coconut milk like this promotes hair growth and if your hair is beginning to turn gray, the new growth will come in with your natural hair color. Even after each treatment you may notice the color of your hair becoming a little richer and darker.

If you like, you could also add a touch of oil after washing your hair. Don't use too much; a few drops will do. Rub it into your hands and then brush your fingers through your hair transferring the oil to your hair and scalp. A few drops will not make your hair look oily, but it is enough to give a little extra luster. After being shampooed, the hair and scalp are usually very dry so a little dab of coconut oil will do it good.

Coconut oil has a long history of use as a hair conditioner in the islands. Those who use it appear to have thick, rich colored hair. What has been observed for centuries is backed by science. Studies have shown that using coconut oil in the hair can help prevent combing damage and improve its health and appearance. An interesting study was reported in the *Journal of Cosmetic Science* on coconut oil's effect on hair health.[1] In this study coconut oil was compared with sunflower oil and mineral oil—the two most extensively used in hair oil formulations. "The findings" as the authors of the study state, "clearly indicate the strong impact coconut oil application has to hair as compared to the application of both sunflower and mineral oils." Among the three oils, coconut oil was the only one that reduced protein loss for both undamaged and damaged hair when used as a pre-wash and post-wash grooming product. Neither sunflower nor mineral oil reduced protein loss in hair. The authors of the study indicated that the difference in results was due to the composition of each of the oils. Coconut oil, being rich in medium-chain triglycerides is able to penetrate inside the hair shaft, protecting it from protein loss, as well as giving it more body. Mineral oil, being a hydrocarbon, has no affinity for proteins and, therefore, is not able to penetrate the hair. In the case of sunflower oil, it is composed of long-chain triglycerides that do not penetrate either, resulting in no favorable impact on protein loss. Since nearly *all* other vegetable and plant oils are composed of long-chain triglycerides, just as sunflower oil is, they too do not protect against protein loss. Only coconut oil can protect the hair from protein loss and prevent hair damage. Therefore, it is the best oil to use for your hair care.

Suntan Oil

Coconut oil is the original suntan lotion. It's been used by generations of happy islanders. At one time it was the main ingredient in commercial suntan and sunscreen lotions and is still used in some brands today.

Coconut oil is the best natural suntan and sunscreen lotion there is. Apply the oil to all exposed surfaces of the skin. Don't use too much or it will pool on the surface of the skin and wipe off on clothing. As I mentioned at the beginning of this chapter, coconut oil gives me several hours of protection from the sun and I am fair-skinned. The effectiveness of coconut oil in protecting you from sunburn, however, depends also on your diet. If you eat or have eaten a diet rich in unsaturated fats (e.g., soybean, corn, canola, safflower oils), you will be more prone to burning. A diet rich in coconut oil and other saturated fats will protect you. Even if you have been eating coconut oil regularly for several weeks or months, if you previously ate a lot of polyunsaturated oils, then your skin will still contain a large amount of polyunsaturated fat which is highly vulnerable to peroxidation and sunburn. It may take several months to replace the oils in your body and in your skin. Go slowly.

As you get sun exposure, your body will adjust by producing more melanin—the dark pigment in the skin that helps protect you from sunburn. If you are not accustomed to getting much sun, I suggest you limit your exposure to about 15 to 20 minutes at first. If your skin becomes red, cut back on the time you spend in the sun. Apply coconut oil on all exposed skin. Use coconut oil liberally in the diet. Avoid all polyunsaturated oils and limit monounsaturated oils. Use coconut oil as your primary source of cooking oil.

Gradually increase the amount of time you spend under the sun. Add 5 or 10 minutes after a week or so. Monitor the redness of your skin. You want to avoid burning. Gradually lengthen out your time until you reach 30 or 60 minutes or however long you want to spend in the sun.

If you know you will be exposed to a great deal of sunlight for some reason, such as going hiking or sailing, you can build up your tolerance to the

Skin, Hair, and Nails

Two months ago I started eating fresh coconuts, one a week, I ate most of the meat. And now, for two weeks virgin coconut oil about a teaspoon a day. My knees and elbows today have smooth skin. All my life they have had rough skin. I can hardly believe it! I am astonished at this improvement in my skin. All my life I can remember rough skin on my knees and elbows. Also, I think my face has less wrinkles.

Lawrence

I have for a long, long time had a painful problem with my heels cracking. (I blame this along with a myriad of other problems on my hypothyroidism.) I decided to rub the coconut oil into my heels. This felt so good that I put it all over my feet, including in and round my toes, after my morning shower. Well, what I have noticed are 2 things: 1) where I had the beginnings of some apparent athlete's foot on one of my little toes, it disappeared in 3 days, and 2) I have no foot odor whatsoever. Oh, and by the way, after a week of rubbing in the oil I no longer had any cracking heels either. My feet still feel like such a novelty to me because I haven't had smooth heels in I don't know how long. Nothing else really helped before, not pumice stones and creams, nothing.

Anna

One of my very favorite, and super simple hair treatments is canned coconut milk. I call this "recipe" a soak because it's really drippy with a thin consistency. Anyway…Apply as much coconut milk (canned and not lite) to your dry hair as your hair will absorb. Make sure to work it in really well. Top it with a shower cap (or plastic bag) and a turban or towel. Apply heat for as long as you can manage (heat cap, hot towel, blow dryer, forced air heating vent). Shampoo out with a gentle shampoo and follow up with your regular conditioner or detangler. Style as usual. Sometimes the easiest things work the best. I love this, plus it smells good.

Stephanie

I went to my doctor (a woman) today and she noticed my hands and arms and commented on how soft they looked and felt! I told her that I've been using coconut oil daily from my face to the bottoms of my feet, after bathing. It is also great for cuticles. I'm no spring chicken either.

Doris

I use virgin coconut oil on my hair. I put it in before bed. I rub it together in my hands and work it through (make sure you get your scalp, too), then brush. Make sure you have a separate brush for this. You wouldn't want to use the same brush for your regular brushing and styling. I leave it in overnight and shampoo and do regular conditioning the next day. My hair feels so smooth and soft you wouldn't believe it. It's a great deep conditioner.

Lori

Since using virgin coconut oil regularly I have noticed my fingernails getting strong as iron. I can hardly chew them anymore and will have to look for a new bad habit.

Elaine

I have thin hair with curl in it and I've noticed it growing much faster and becoming stronger/thicker since starting on the oil 2 months ago. My nails are also growing. They were brittle and barely grew at all prior to coconut oil, always breaking and splitting. I cannot believe the difference in my nails since starting to take the oil. AMAZING!

Megan

I have been using coconut oil on my skin and a little in my hair for shine for about 6 months now. It appears to be very good for it. Rough places like my elbows have become so soft...To me it seems almost like it's a vitamin for my skin. It just looks so much healthier. My skin tone has evened out and it's smooth and healthier than it's been in a long time.

Tish

My husband has been using coconut oil in his hair for a year now and his hair is definitely thicker and has more of it on the top of his head where he was receding a bit. He was just using it like a hair gel, not knowing of this other benefit.

Suzanne

My athlete's foot fungus, which used to be very irritating, has gone very quiet. This seems to be attributable to internal action by the coconut oil. I have used no other medication of any sort but am really amazed at how the problem disappeared.

Mike

sun this way. A daily 30 minute sunbath is enough to prepare yourself. When you go on your trip apply coconut oil and reapply as often as you feel it is needed. I rarely apply it more than once or twice unless the oil is washed off. If you follow these guidelines, you won't have a problem even if you spend several hours in the sun.

Injuries and Infections

Coconut will speed the healing of all types of injuries and infections and will prevent ugly scarring. If applied before the injury occurs, healing will be faster. This is one good reason to use it daily. As an example, if coconut oil is massaged into the abdomen of an expectant mother and continued after delivery, stretch marks won't be a problem. Body builders sometimes complain that as they beef up they develop stretch marks. This problem can be avoided with daily use of coconut oil both topically and internally. Cuts, burns, and other injuries heal faster and with less scarring if treated with coconut oil.

Injuries, infections, growths (warts and moles), and blemishes of every kind respond very well to coconut oil therapy. Warm the oil first. Put the container in hot water until the oil is very warm, not just lukewarm. Warm oil is absorbed more efficiently and penetrates deeper. When applying the oil, it is best to massage or work the oil into the skin. Massaging the oil into the skin also increases absorption. If you have an injury you might not be able to do this. Brushing on a light coat may be as much as you can do.

The secret to getting the best results with coconut oil is to keep it continually on the injured or infected spot until healed. You can do this using a bandage. If you can't use a bandage, you should apply the oil as frequently as possible throughout the day.

With a bandage you can keep the infected or injured spot continually in contact with the oil. You want to keep the bandage moist all the time. That doesn't mean it needs to be dripping wet, just wet enough to allow the skin to continually absorb the oil. The bandage should be kept this way day and night until the injury is healed.

Ordinary Band-Aids don't work well. After several hours the oil tends to dissolve the adhesive and they slip off. A piece of cloth, plastic wrap, and adhesive tape or an elastic band can work. Cut a piece of cloth or gauze so it is a little larger than the injured area on the skin. Take a piece of plastic wrap or plastic sandwich bag and cut it so that it is about a half inch or so larger than the cloth. Soak the cloth in melted coconut oil. Rub some warm oil into the skin. Wipe off excess oil around the injury. The skin around the injury must be oil-free to allow the tape to stick to the skin. Apply the oil-soaked cloth to the injury. Lay the plastic on top of the cloth. Secure the cloth and plastic with the adhesive tape or an elastic band. The purpose of the plastic is to keep the oil from soaking into the tape and onto your clothes and bed sheets. Add more oil as needed to keep the bandage moist. Replace the bandage with a new one every day.

You can use a commercial bandage in place of the one described above, if you can find one that works. The most effective and convenient bandage I have found is a product made by 3M called Tegaderm. It's made of hypoallergenic,

---

Insect Bites

Let me tell you I have become a very firm believer. The other day I accidentally stepped into a nest of fire ants. For anyone that has never had contact with these little devils, let me tell you they are correctly named. They are vicious little creatures and the bites they inflict burn like fire. I had on sandals and before I could step out of the nest many had bitten all over my bare feet and ankles. The bites immediately began to burn like fire. I went inside to get something to put on the bites and thought about the virgin coconut oil. Why not try it? I smeared it all over my ankles and feet where I had been bitten. I am amazed and so is my husband. The burning stopped right away and the bites are tiny and almost gone within 2 days, and no itching. The amazing part is I have had these ant bites several times before and nothing I put on stopped the burning or itching that comes afterward. The bites would grow huge and fill with puss and last for days.

Barbara

Mosquitoes no longer are just considered a pesty summer nuisance but also come bearing the threat of West Nile Virus. As much as I hate the thought of having to spray myself down with Deep Woods Off every time I go outside in the early morning or dusk hours of the day wearing shorts and tank tops, I do it. Well 98% of the time anyways. On the 2 occasions lately when I have been out and forgotten to spray down I have been eaten alive by the little buggers. The histamines immediately kick in and the bites swell and itch like crazy! The first time it happened I fortunately had a small jar of melted virgin coconut oil in my truck (it was 93 degrees that day) and I thought well it seems to be the miracle cure for everything else let's see what it will do for mosquito bites! I rubbed it into all of my bites and believe it or not, not only did it stop the itch, but within 30 minutes all of the bites were flat!! Last night I had the opportunity to try it out again and had the same results!! This morning there are no traces of any mosquito bites!!! Is this stuff GREAT or what??!!!

Sharyn

The photo at left shows a close-up of the right index finger, illustrating the condition of skin prior to using coconut oil. The skin is severely dry and rough. The picture on the right is the same finger after using coconut oil for three weeks.

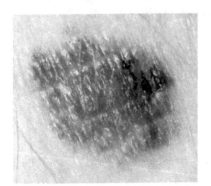 

Photo on left shows a melanoma, an aggressive form of skin cancer. Coconut oil was applied topically every few days and the melanoma noticeably began to fade within a couple of months. After a year the melanoma was completely gone, right photo.

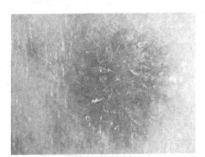 

Photo on left shows a scar left by a deep bruise that persisted for four years without showing any signs of fading. Coconut oil was massaged into the injury almost daily and within a couple of months most of the scarring had faded, right photo.

166

non-latex material that is breathable and self-adhesive. It comes in various sizes, but you can cut it into smaller sizes or odd shapes if you like. Tegaderm takes the place of the plastic wrap and adhesive tape described above. You will still need to use a piece of cloth soaked in the oil. Tegaderm holds the cloth in place without the oil leaking or making a mess. Look for it at your local pharmacy or medical supply store. If the stores in your area don't have it, you can contact the company directly by calling (USA) 1-800-228-3957.

If the affected area is on your hands, it can be difficult to wear a bandage without it falling off. A simple way to solve this problem is to put the oil on your hand and cover it with an inexpensive cellophane glove. Wear it to bed and remove it in the morning. Repeat each night until the condition improves.

Please note that commercial creams and lotions containing coconut oil, although good, do not have the healing power of pure coconut oil. If you want to see quick improvement, use coconut oil rather than creams and lotions.

Sickness

Normally if you feel sick, eating some coconut oil can help you feel better. Sometimes, however, you may not be able to take coconut oil orally. You may be nauseous or vomiting. You can still benefit from the oil by massaging it into the body. Because of their small size, MCTs are easily absorbed into the skin. For this reason, they are often used as carriers in delivering medications in transdermal patches that are applied to the skin. Likewise, coconut oil is easily absorbed into the skin and into the bloodstream. So you can still get some benefit simply by applying it topically.

Generally, if you have an illness that does not prevent you from eating, you can attack the problem from two angles—internally and externally. Add

---

Warts

I started using it about a month ago on my skin (I have very dry and sensitive skin). I had some places on the back of my legs and the tops of my feet that have had tiny warts on them and within 1 week, they all fell off!!!! My skin is smooth, not cracked. I didn't use it on my face at first thinking it's oil and I would get blemishes (acne) from it. I was wrong in my thinking. I got one of those deep blemishes, on my chin and put it on and the pain and bump were gone the next day. I now use it on my face and my skin is flawless! I have had my teenage son use it on his face instead of his prescription acne cream and his face is clear! I also now have long fingernails. They used to always crack and peel and now they are strong and hard.

Robin

---

coconut oil to your food and massage it into your skin. It is recommended that you apply warm oil to the skin closest to the infected area. Use warm oil because it gets better penetration. If you have a chest cold, for example, rub the oil into the chest and back and along the neck. If the feet are numb, rub the oil there. Whichever part of the body needs help, that's where you apply the oil.

USING COCONUT INTERNALLY
Maintenance Dose

One of the first questions people ask when they learn about the benefits of coconut oil is how much they should use each day. The simple answer to that question is: any amount that you feel comfortable with. Even a half a teaspoon taken daily is beneficial. Paul Sorse only took one teaspoon daily, but he also absorbed another couple of tablespoons through his skin and ate fresh coconut and coconut milk. For a person who weighed less than 120 pounds, he received a healthy dose of oil.

The general recommendation is 3½ tablespoons a day for an average-sized adult. This value is derived from the amount of medium-chain fatty acids nature puts in human breast milk. The amount infants receive protects them from infectious illness and provides adequate nutritional support under normal circumstances. Based on ideal body size, a 150-pound adult should consume 3½ tablespoons of coconut oil to equal the amount of MCFAs an infant receives.

For most people 3 to 4 tablespoons a day is ample. If you weigh less than 150 pounds at your ideal weight, subtract ½ tablespoon for each 25 pounds under this weight. For those who are larger than 150 pounds, 4 tablespoons is generally plenty. See table below.

Suggested Daily Dose	
Body Weight (lb/kg)	Tablespoons of Oil
175+/79+	4
150/68	3½
125/57	3
100/45	2½
75/34	2
50/23	1½
25/11	1

The above table is only a general guideline; it is not an absolute rule. Many people experience wonderful results with only 1 tablespoon a day. Keep in mind that *any* amount is beneficial. It's perfectly okay to get a little more or less and for the amount to fluctuate some from day to day.

You can consume the oil in any manner that is convenient for you. Some people take the oil by the spoonful like a dietary supplement. Others mix it with juice or food. For most people I recommend that you take it with food. Many people do not like eating oil straight from a spoon. Some people may even have a gag reflex trying to swallow any type of oil. The easiest way to get your daily dose is by using the oil in your food preparation. Use coconut oil in place of other oils.

I also recommend you do not consume all of the oil at one time. Spread it out over the entire day or at least divide it in half, taking some at one meal and some at another. Also take into account the amount of oil you get from other coconut products—meat and milk.

Therapeutic Dose

In most cases, even when you are sick, 3½ tablespoons of oil per day is generally adequate. However, the antimicrobial effects of MCFAs are accumulative, so the more you have in your body the more effective they are in fighting off infections. You can take as much as twice the maintenance dose if you feel the need. Some doctors recommend 6 or more tablespoons a day for their very sick patients. Don't take this amount all at once. A tablespoon or so taken every 2 to 3 hours is a good schedule to follow. Too much oil, any oil, if you're not accustomed to it will give you loose stools, so spread the amount throughout the day and eat it with a little food or a beverage.

There is no danger of overdosing on coconut oil. Coconut oil is a food, not a drug. Human populations have consumed twice as much as the maintenance dose for years with no adverse effects. I know people working on serious health problems that were taking 10 to 14 tablespoons a day and experienced no adverse side effects. I have personally taken up to 14 tablespoons daily for several days without problem. If you take more than your body can handle, the worst symptoms you might experience are a runny stool and perhaps intestinal uneasiness for a time. To avoid this, simply reduce the amount of oil. Also, if you eat the oil with a good source of soluble fiber, like psyllium husk, you will have less trouble with nausea and loose stools.

If you cannot consume the oil or any other food because of nausea or vomiting, apply the oil topically to the area that is most affected as described earlier. At least this way you will get some benefit from the oil. If you do not have problems consuming the oil when you are sick, it is a good idea to take advantage of the oil's healing properties both internally and externally. Massage the oil into the skin as well as eat it. This will give you double benefit.

Adding Coconut to Your Diet

So how do you add coconut oil to your diet? The easiest way is to simply replace all your other oils with coconut oil. Replace coconut oil in recipes that call for margarine, shortening, butter, or vegetable oil. In most cases you can replace the equivalent amount of coconut oil for these other oils.

Many people take the oil on a daily basis by the tablespoon. You can do this easily with a good quality oil that has a delicate coconut taste. Most people, however, just can't handle taking oil, any oil straight from the spoon. You don't need to eat it by the spoon. Try taking it with a beverage. Add a tablespoon of oil to hot cocoa, herbal tea, or juice. The beverage needs to be warm or hot so that the oil remains liquid. If you pour melted coconut oil into a cup of cold orange juice, it will form lumps. So juice needs to be warmed. Hot tomato juice and coconut oil go well together. It tastes like a soup. Most beverages are water-based so the oil will float to the top; just stir and drink quickly.

Coconut oil can be added to many dishes. Use it as a spread on bread, a topping on vegetables, add it to pasta, casseroles, soups, and stews. It goes well mixed into hot cereal. Use it for all your cooking and baking needs.

You don't have to restrict yourself to eating just coconut oil to get MCFAs. Coconut meat and milk also contain them. Eating a piece of fresh coconut or drinking a beverage made with coconut milk may suit your tastes better than swallowing a spoonful of oil. Adding these other coconut products into your diet is a pleasant way of getting your daily dose of coconut oil.

How much oil do you get from coconut meat and milk? To get 3½ tablespoons of oil you need 7 ounces of fresh mature coconut (about half

OIL CONTENT OF COCONUT MILK

Coconut milk(oz)	Oil (Tbsp)
1	½
2	¾
3	1
4	1½
5	1¾
6	2
7	2½
8	2¾
9	3
10	3½

Oil values are rounded off to the nearest quarter tablespoon.
Values are based on full-fat milk, not light or reduced fat coconut milk, containing10 grams of fat per 2 ounce (59 ml) serving.

a coconut), 2¾ cups dried coconut, or 10 ounces of coconut milk. Eating half a coconut a day may be a bit difficult for most people, but drinking 10 ounces of coconut milk is rather easy. Three ounces of coconut milk provides approximately 1 tablespoon of oil.

Coconut meat has its own health benefits due to its high fiber content. Fresh coconut makes an excellent low-calorie snack. Shredded or grated coconut goes well with fruit salads, smoothies, and baked goods. Coconut flour can be used in place of, or in addition to, other flours in making breads and casseroles. Coconut flour can be added to juices, smoothies, and baked goods to increase fiber intake.

Coconut milk is very versatile and can be used to make a wide variety of foods such as chowders, smoothies, salad dressings, and sauces. It makes a great replacement for cow's milk and is excellent in baked goods. If you are interested in learning how to add coconut into your diet I highly recommend that you get a copy of my *Coconut Miracle Cookbook*. This book contains nearly 450 recipes using coconut oil, meat, milk, and cream. Dishes include salads, beverages, soups and chowders, main dishes, side dishes, and desserts.

GETTING THE BEST RESULTS

Many people can testify that coconut in one form or another has significantly changed their lives for the better. Some have found relief after suffering for years with chronic health problems. Some of the stories told by these people are truly remarkable. For these people coconut has worked miracles.

There are also people who try coconut products for a while but for some reason don't experience the noticeable changes that others have. Why is it that for some people coconut is a miracle worker and for others it's not? There are several likely reasons.

One of the pitfalls we often fall into after finding a product that can do so much is to think it can do anything and everything. Let me be the first one to tell you that coconut isn't a cure-all. Coconut can work wonders but it can't cure everything. Coconut oil, for example, is a powerful antimicrobial, but it won't kill all disease-causing germs. The common cold virus, for example, is not directly affected by it. This doesn't mean coconut oil can't help you when you have a cold. The oil does aid the immune system so in that respect it can be of benefit. Although coconut oil and other coconut products may not be effective in treating every health problem, its use certainly won't do any harm and you shouldn't be afraid of using it.

Another reason people don't get the results they want is that they often don't give it a fair chance. They don't use it long enough to see a difference. Coconut is not a drug and you cannot expect it to bring about immediate results like some drugs do. Unlike drugs, coconut is a food and, therefore, supports the body's own natural healing processes. It provides the building blocks—vitamins, minerals, phytonutrients, medium-chain fatty acids—that help the body fight off disease, repair damaged tissues, and maintain proper physiological functions. You cannot expect chronic health problems that have been present for many years to vanish overnight. A problem that has endured for 10 years isn't usually going to go away in a few days or weeks. It may take months or even years to correct some problems. Coconut in itself isn't a cure for any particular disease or health problem. What it does is provide the body with the nutritional elements it needs to heal itself. You have to wait for the body to do the healing. Sometimes this can take a while.

The speed at which the body heals is determined to a great extent by your diet and lifestyle. The old adage "You are what you eat" is very true. Our cells and tissues are built from the foods we eat. If we eat poor quality foods lacking in essential nutrients, our bodies cannot build healthy bones, muscles, and tissues. It's just like a contractor building a house: if he uses cheap materials, the house will deteriorate and fall apart quickly. In like manner, if we feed our bodies poor quality foods, our bodies will be weak and susceptible to disease.

One woman commented, "I was disillusioned when I first started taking coconut oil." She had heard so much good about the oil that she was discouraged when she wasn't seeing a quick recovery. It was not until she increased the amount of oil she took and cut out sugar and refined flour and all processed foods that she started feeling the benefits of the oil. "I also began losing weight though I was eating more fat." She adds, "Remember that though coconut oil is a miracle food, it cannot make miracles happen without other changes in the diet." Well said.

Coconut products provide an excellent source of nutrition, fiber, and other elements that promote better health and ward off disease, but they can't make up for a poor diet. If you live on donuts and coffee, you will develop health problems. No amount of coconut added to the diet will compensate for dietary abuse. Coconut can help, even when the diet is poor, but to achieve the best results, to experience the "miracles" that others have, you need to eat properly. Those who complain that coconut doesn't help them are usually the ones who eat the worst types of foods and expect coconut to act like a wonder drug. The healthier your diet is, the faster coconut will aid you in overcoming health problems.

When it comes to dietary advice it seems that everyone has his or her own opinion. Even the so-called nutritional experts don't agree. Some promote vegetarianism or raw-foodism while others promote high-protein diets. One expert will say low-fat, high-carbohydrate diets are the way to go while another will claim a moderate or high-fat, low-carbohydrate diet is better. And still others will say we should base our dietary choices on metabolism or blood type. Opinions often run strong as to which is more correct.

I'm not going to attempt to recommend any particular diet in this book. What I am going to do is make some general recommendations that would be compatible with almost any of these diets. When you look at all the different diets, you find that people have benefited from most of them. Even those that seem to be complete opposites such as vegetarianism (low meat and fat intake) and low-carbohydrate diets (high meat and fat intake) have proven to be successful. Why is that? One reason I believe is that they try to eliminate poor quality foods and focus on the eating the healthiest ones. Regardless of what type of diet you prefer, if you follow the simple guidelines below you will do okay.

The foods you should avoid:
Overly processed grains (white flour, white bread, white rice, breakfast cereal, crackers, etc.)
Sugar and sweets (candy, cookies, desserts, soda, etc.)
Pasteurized and homogenized milk
Processed vegetable oils
Hydrogenated vegetable oils (margarine and shortening)

The foods you should eat more of:
Fresh fruits and vegetables

Most of us do not eat nearly enough fresh fruits and vegetables. Studies continually show that fruits and particularly vegetables contain nutrients that help protect us from disease and retard aging. The standard recommendation is that we get at least (a bare minimum) of 5 servings of fruits and vegetables a day. Some researchers are now recommending that we get 9 or more servings a day, mostly vegetables. You should not *add* more food to your diet but *replace* the breads, grains, and refined and processed foods with the additional servings of vegetables, both raw and cooked. Vegetables should provide the bulk of your diet, complemented by other healthy foods. If you follow this simple piece of dietary advice you will have a fairly healthy diet.

I like the quote from noted author and nutritionist Dr. Gabriel Cousens: "With the proper diet, no doctor is necessary. With the improper diet, no doctor can help." If you eat properly when you start using coconut products you will see rapid improvement. If you don't see improvement then you should re-evaluate your diet. The recommendations above are only basic guidelines. There are many other foods in the diet that do not promote good health. These include: coffee, alcohol, food additives (preservatives, flavor enhancers, dyes, etc.), dehydrated/powdered cheese and eggs, and artificial sweeteners. If you don't see the results you expected, you should probably reevaluate your diet.

Aches and Pains

I can't quite imagine that virgin coconut oil would help my hip bursitis, but within less than a week the pain level had diminished vastly! I had such pain that I was taking 4 Ibuprofen every 4-5 hours. At night I could only sleep on one side and that hurt. I had to use a heat pad to get any relief so I could sleep. I am off the pills and the heat pad.

Gerri

The pain that I get in my shoulder from sleeping on one side for more than 2 hours is pretty much gone. The pain from stretching my arm across my chest, which I have had for at least 10 years, is GONE. It is amazing.

Roger

I have what was diagnosed 1½ years ago as a degenerative disk in my lower back. Bone-on-bone which was so painful I had to lie on a heating pad every night when I came home from work and had trouble sitting and lying down. Standing was the only relief. The physical therapist did not help. The painkillers helped but my doctor wouldn't renew the prescription, said surgery would be my last resort so I best just learn to live with it and change my lifestyle. [I began using coconut oil and] about a month ago the pain started to subside and now I am virtually pain free.

Rox

For several months I have been experiencing some pain with swelling in one of my knees. Upon receipt of the expeller pressed coconut oil I began taking 2 teaspoons a day to see how it would react with me. I also began rubbing my knee with the expeller pressed coconut oil and for the past 2 or 3 days I have not experienced any pain or swelling in that knee.

Chris

My husband has regained complete use of his shoulders and his joints are pain free for the first time in over 12 years. He takes about 1-2 tablespoons of coconut oil in his coffee every morning. He has lost 15 pounds and noticed an increase in energy the first day he took the coconut oil.

Belinda

In treating serious illnesses or chronic disease, using coconut and making wise dietary choices may not be enough. You may need other forms of treatment as well. In this case you should seek the counsel of an experienced health care professional.

PRECAUTIONS WITH COCONUT
Side Effects

Is coconut safe? If the MCFAs in coconut oil are powerful enough to kill bacteria, viruses, and parasites, couldn't they harm us as well? One of the most often asked questions I hear is how safe is it? How much can you eat? Are there any side effects? Consider this: nature puts MCFAs in mother's breast milk. If it is safe enough for a newborn infant, it should be safe enough for anyone else. The fact that it is in breast milk attests to its safety.

Coconut oil has been maligned for so long that many people hesitate to use any coconut product for fear it might harm them. Even when they have seen the evidence of the benefits some still wonder if there are any harmful side effects. Let me put your fears at ease. There are no harmful side effects to using coconut oil or any other coconut product. Dr. Jon Kabara who has done research on coconut for over half a century agrees. He states, "Fatty acids and derivatives tend to be the least toxic chemicals known to man. Not only are these agents nontoxic to man but are actual foods."[2]

Coconut is a food. If you are not allergic to it you should be able to eat it without problem. One effect, however, and it depends on how you look at it, is that consuming *too much* coconut oil or coconut water can loosen the bowels. If you are troubled by constipation this may be a good thing. If you consume the oil and water along with other foods, and not by themselves, the effect is greatly reduced. As your body becomes accustomed to coconut products this effect will lessen.

Allergies and Food Sensitivities

Some people report that when they start using coconut oil externally or internally, their skin breaks out in a rash. This reaction could be a response to one of two things. It could be a cleansing reaction, and the body is expelling toxins, or it could be an allergic reaction to coconut.

If you have trouble with allergies, before using any coconut product you may want to test yourself to see if you might be allergic to it. People can be allergic or hypersensitive to any type of food, even broccoli or lettuce. Some people are allergic to coconut. A simple way to test yourself is to put a little coconut oil or milk on your forearm. Rub it into the skin. Wait a day and see what happens. If the skin becomes red or swollen, you may be allergic; if nothing happens you probably aren't. You will know if you are allergic or not with just one application.

Even if you are allergic to most nuts, you are not likely to be allergic to coconut. Coconut is considered to be a low allergy risk food and a true allergy to coconut is rare. For the person who has food allergies, and is not allergic to coconut, coconut products may provide a safe and tasty alternative. Coconut milk and other coconut products can be used in a surprising variety of ways from delicate desserts to hearty main courses. Coconut meat can be used in place of nuts in most recipes, and coconut milk makes an excellent replacement for cow's milk. Coconut milk and cream are good for making rich, creamy smoothies, chowders, cream pies, puddings, and even ice cream.

Healing Crisis

Occasionally people will complain that coconut, particularly coconut oil, makes them constipated while others will say it gives them diarrhea. Some claim it causes their skin to break out or produce any number of other symptoms. They assume they are allergic to coconut or that it just doesn't agree with them.

Ordinarily, when you start doing things that are supposed to be good for you, you would expect to feel better. However, this is not always the case. Sometimes you may get worse before you get better, a surprising and confusing result to many people.

Certain healing foods, herbs, and nutritional supplements can exert a powerful influence on the body by accelerating the processes of detoxification and regeneration. At times this cleansing and rebuilding process can become so intense that a number of symptoms appear. This period of intense cleaning is called a "healing crisis." It is referred to as a "crisis" because it involves somewhat unpleasant symptoms such as fatigue and nausea. It is regarded as "healing" because the body is experiencing an accelerated period of cleansing and healing. Although a healing crisis may make you feel like you are ill, it is not an illness and you should not be afraid of it.

Physicians experienced in using diet and other natural, drug-less therapies often see patients go through healing crises. In fact, a healing crisis is a sign that treatment is working and patients are encouraged to look forward to it.

Coconut oil has an incredible healing quality that can initiate a healing crisis. A cleansing reaction can occur whether you use the oil internally or externally. When I first started massaging my whole body with the oil, I noticed that I had an increase in acne. I would get pimples on my legs and stomach—places I don't normally get acne. It wasn't a whole lot, maybe one or two a week. Normally I'm rarely troubled with acne, so it was very unusual and noticeable. At first, I wondered if it was the particular brand of oil I was using. Perhaps, I thought, the oil had impurities, dirt or something, that was causing the acne. I tried another brand that was processed differently, but the same thing happened. So it seemed to be a characteristic of the oil and not something to do with the processing. After a month or so the acne problem went away. Since then I've had no problem with acne.

Later, other people reported similar experiences. I wasn't alone. It confirmed my suspicion. The oil was penetrating the skin, helping the body rid itself of impurities. The acne was just the body's way of cleansing itself. So don't worry about acne when you use coconut oil; it will go away when the skin has cleaned itself out. In fact, many people find that coconut oil helps clear up acne.

Anything that stimulates the body's own recuperative powers has the potential to cause a healing crisis. As the body gets stronger and healthier, it will reach a level where it can sustain a period of intense cleansing and rebuilding. At this point, the body becomes strong enough to pull out and remove toxins, germs, and diseased tissues, many of which could have been buried for years. These poisons are pulled out of the tissues and dumped into the bloodstream, to be removed through the body's channels of elimination. As these toxins are purged from the body, symptoms of elimination become manifest. Common symptoms include fatigue, nausea, vomiting, diarrhea, skin rashes, acne, headaches, muscle aches and pains, loss of appetite, fever, depression, and mood swings, to mention just a few. *Any* type of symptom can be associated with a healing crisis.

Those who go through a healing crisis won't necessarily experience all of these symptoms, maybe only one or two at a time. Because we all have different genes, diets, and lifestyles, the symptoms one person may experience will be different from those of another. The severity of the symptoms usually depends on the level of health of the individual. Those who are in poor health will have more severe symptoms than those who are in better health. Symptoms may be so severe that you will want to stay in bed for a day or two, or they may be so mild you won't even notice them. Generally, a healing crisis will only last a couple of days, but sometimes it may persist for a week or more. In some cases a reaction may occur each time a healing substance (such a coconut) is consumed until the body has been able to reach a higher state of health.

I recommend that people start off slowly when adding coconut products into the diet. This is especially true for coconut oil. Don't start taking 3½ tablespoons of oil all at once or even all in one day. Many people after learning of the wonderful benefits of coconut oil jump in headfirst and gulp down 3 or 4 tablespoons at once. If your body isn't accustomed to eating this much oil or if you have some serious health issues, you could experience some unpleasant symptoms or discomfort. For this reason I recommend that you start off with one tablespoon a day taken with food. If you have no problems, then use two tablespoons and gradually work up to a maintenance dose. Take a small amount throughout the day rather than one large single dose. Three teaspoons equals one tablespoon. Try taking 1 teaspoon three times a day, and eat it with food.

In this book, when I talk about teaspoons and tablespoons I am not referring to the spoons you use for eating but the actual measurement of a teaspoon or tablespoon. One tablespoon equals 15 ml and 1 teaspoon equals 5 ml. Two tablespoons equals 1 fluid ounce.

For some people even a single teaspoon will cause the runs. This suggests that there is a problem with the digestive system. It's not the oil that is causing the problem; it's the reaction of a troubled digestive system adjusting to the oil. If you find you can only tolerate a teaspoon or two, stay at that dosage. As your body becomes stronger and more accustomed to the oil, you can increase the dosage. A healthy person should have no adverse reactions to 3½ tablespoons of coconut oil. Coconut meat and oil support digestive health and help to balance the intestinal environment.

Keep in mind that the symptoms associated with a healing crisis are processes that facilitate healing. If you experience diarrhea, for example, it means your body is eliminating toxins through the bowels. Let the symptoms run their course. There is nothing to fear from a healing crisis. It is not an illness and you need not take any medications to relieve symptoms. In fact, taking medications will suppress the symptoms and stop the cleansing process.

As your health improves you may go through several healing crises. Each one may be accompanied by different symptoms. With each crisis your health is elevated to a higher level. You will gradually feel better and better. For a more in-depth discussion of the healing crisis, how to recognize it, and what to do when it comes, I recommend my book *The Healing Crisis*.

The Real Danger of Coconut:
Neurological Damage?

Coconut is one of the safest foods you can eat; it's hypoallergenic and has no harmful side effects. However, there is one caution you should be aware of, especially if you live where coconuts are plentiful. Those people who live in the coconut growing regions of the world have a much higher incidence of coconut-induced brain injuries. This is a fact. Doctors agree that the greatest harm a coconut can do to you is fall out of a tree and hit you on your head. It has been reported that despite its superior nutritional properties, a hard heavy coconut can deliver a powerful impact when dropped out of a 100-foot tree. A single coconut can deliver a metric ton of force. That's enough power to dent even the hardest skull.

According to Peter Barss of McGill University in Canada, falling coconuts can produce "really severe, sometimes fatal neural injuries: by hitting an artery and causing bleeding inside the skull." When he worked in a hospital in Papua

New Guinea he found that falling coconuts caused 2.5 percent of all trauma admissions. For this reason, many urban areas have cut down their coconut trees to avoid this danger.

Dr. Barss admits that more injuries come from people falling out of trees than from falling coconuts. Fortunately, this health problem occurs only in the tropics and rarely at that. If you live outside the tropics, your chances of being hit by a falling coconut are zero.

What can we conclude from this? There is a far greater danger in standing next to a coconut palm than there is in eating a coconut. So enjoy using coconut. Make it a part of your life. It may just be your key to happiness, health, and beauty.

Chapter 8

PROCEDURES, FORMULAS, AND RECIPES

If you are like most people, especially if you live outside coconut country, you probably have no idea how to use coconut or how to distinguish a good quality coconut from a not-so-good one. In this chapter you will become familiar with identifying quality coconuts and coconut products and how to use them. You will learn how to make your own coconut milk, cream, oil, and shredded meat from fresh coconut. You will find directions for making homemade antibacterial coconut soap and rich lathering coconut shampoo. You will also be instructed on how to make coconut-based health foods, tonics, and ointments.

WORKING WITH FRESH COCONUT
How To Choose A Good Coconut

Whole unopened coconuts are available at most grocery stores and in Asian markets. Not all of these coconuts, however, are fit to eat. If you've ever purchased an imported coconut you know what I mean. Once opened, they can smell and taste awful. Unfortunately, if you're not accustomed to eating fresh coconut you may think these poor quality nuts to be the norm. They're not. Fresh, unadulterated coconut is delicious and has a pleasant, mild aroma. Many imported coconuts are old, damaged or moldy, and taste terrible.

Finding a good quality coconut takes a little detective work. Some stores have better coconuts than others so you may want to shop around. This, however, is no guarantee that you will get a good coconut every time as the quality can vary greatly even in the same store. The age of the coconuts and how they are handled affects quality. Coconuts that have been battered around and cracked spoil very quickly. Once a crack occurs in the shell, mold quickly develops

180

inside. Most coconuts are shipped long distances over extended periods of time. You have no way of telling how old they are when you buy them. The older they are the more likely they are to be moldy.

You can identify mold when you break open the coconut and see yellow or brown coloring in the meat or smell an off odor. Sometimes you can smell mold on the outside of the coconut before breaking it open.

When choosing a whole coconut, look for one without any cracks. If the coconut is damp or has wet spots, the shell is probably cracked and the coconut water is leaking. Shake the coconut to detect the swishing sound of the coconut water. If there is little or no water in the coconut, it is old. Avoid those with white spots, particularly around the "eyes." The white is mold that has probably developed from water leaking from a tiny crack.

Even after you follow these guidelines there is no guarantee that you won't get a moldy coconut. But at least your chances of getting a decent one are greatly increased. After you buy a coconut and bring it home, don't leave it on the countertop; store it in the refrigerator. The older it gets, the more likely it will go bad. So keep it refrigerated and eat it as soon as possible.

Even after choosing a coconut with care you may still find once you get home that the one you've chosen contains mold. A little mold is harmless. You need not worry about inadvertently eating a coconut that may have a small amount of mold. Many coconuts will have a spot or two of mold beginning to develop. If the area is small, simply cut it off. The rest of the coconut should be fine. If it tastes bad, however, throw the whole thing away.

Some people are hypersensitive to mold and may have an adverse reaction. This is generally evidenced by an upset stomach after consuming contaminated coconut meat or water. Older coconuts are more likely to contain mold. But any coconut can possibly have mold, even young immature coconuts.

How To Open A Coconut

The mature hard coconuts usually sold in grocery stores can be difficult to crack. In the tropics coconuts are usually opened by hitting them smartly on the equator with the back of a large knife or machete. If done correctly, the coconut will split into two somewhat equal halves. The shells on these coconuts are very resilient and can withstand a great deal of force. It takes a little practice and a few good hard blows with a machete to crack one open. If you're not accustomed to opening a coconut this way, it's best not to even try or you may wind up losing a few fingers.

Another way to open a coconut is to use a hammer. First, puncture *two* of the "eyes" and drain the water. Coconuts have three eyes. One of the eyes is soft and very easy to puncture, the other two are a bit more difficult. I use an ice pick. You may also use a hammer and nail. After draining the liquid, hold the coconut securely on a hard surface, such as a cement floor, and hit it with a hammer. Coconut shells are very hard so you will need to put some force into it and hit it several times. This may not be a good thing to do on your kitchen counter top.

Another, simpler way to crack a coconut shell after draining the water is to place the coconut on a baking sheet and heat it in the oven for 20 minutes at 400 degrees F (200 C). Generally this is enough to loosen the meat and crack the shell. Tap it with a hammer to break off the shell. It should break apart easily.

Break the shell up into several pieces. With a table knife pry the meat away from the shell. The meat will have a thin brown skin or layer on it where it was in contact with the shell. You can trim this off with a vegetable peeler if you like, but it is safe to eat. I find it easier just to leave it on. If you see any brown or yellow discoloration in the white meat, it is mold. Small patches of mold can be cut off and discarded. Most mature coconuts will have a spot or two. If a lot of discoloration is present, throw the whole thing out.

Fresh coconut makes a wonderful snack. Generally, dried coconut is used in most recipes, and the form in which packaged coconut is sold. Coconut is dried to extend shelf life. Drying does not alter its nutritional value. Only water is removed. Dried coconut will remain edible for a couple of months. It is a good idea, however, to keep it refrigerated or frozen.

You can dry freshly grated coconut in a dehydrator or put it in on a cookie sheet in the oven for a couple of hours at low heat. Store unused coconut in an airtight container in the refrigerator. Fresh coconut spoils quickly so eat it within about five days. If you store it in the freezer, it will last about six months.

KNOW YOUR COCONUT OIL
The Different Types of Oil

I know people who say they love the taste of coconut oil while others say they hate it. I find that most of those who don't like coconut oil have only tried cheap, poor quality brands. Even I don't like these brands and wouldn't touch them. If you're going to be using the oil often, you need to use something you enjoy eating. Before you start using coconut oil, you need to learn how to select a quality product.

Coconut oil is processed and produced in a variety of ways that can affect its quality, appearance, and flavor. Because of the number of brands available, shopping for coconut oil can be confusing. Some are labeled "organic" or "expeller pressed," others "virgin," and still others "extra virgin." Some simply say "coconut oil." Which one is the best? Which is healthiest? Which has the highest medium-chain fatty acid content? Does it even matter?

There are basically only two types of coconut oil: RBD and virgin. All others are just versions of these two. The difference between them depends on the amount of processing the oil undergoes and the type of coconut used. The most commonly used oil in food processing and cosmetics is RBD, which stands for "refined, bleached, and deodorized." This oil has undergone extensive processing. The resulting product is colorless, tasteless, and odorless just like most other processed vegetable oils. RBD oil is typically made from dried coconut known as copra. Copra is dried in furnaces, or more typically, laid out in the sun for several weeks. The dried coconut is separated from the shell and the oil is extracted and refined.

The term "virgin" signifies an oil that has been subjected to less intense refining, that usually means lower temperatures and without chemicals. Unlike RBD oils, virgin coconut oil is made from *fresh* coconuts, not copra. The oil is extracted by any number of methods—boiling, fermentation, refrigeration, mechanical press, or centrifuge. Since high temperatures and chemical solvents are not used, the oil retains its naturally occurring phytochemicals (plant chemicals), which produce a distinctive, yet mild, coconut flavor and aroma.

One term that has caused confusion is "extra virgin" coconut oil. Some manufacturers add the word "extra" to indicate that their virgin oil was processed without any added heat, making it a raw food, which some customers prefer. The problem is that there is no law that prohibits the use of this term for heat-treated virgin oils. Consequently, some brands of coconut oil that have been processed with added heat incorrectly use this term on their products as a marketing gimmick. The only way to tell if the oil is truly raw is by the taste and smell. Raw oils will have a sweet, delicate coconut flavor and aroma. Heat-treated oils often have a slight roasted or cooked flavor.

Another term you're likely to encounter in respect to coconut oil is "expeller pressed." This is a common term used in the vegetable oil industry to describe oils that have had minimal processing. Expeller pressed coconut oil has undergone more processing than virgin oils but not as much as RBD oils. Such oils may be made from either fresh coconut or copra.

Virgin coconut oil made from fresh coconut is a pure white when the oil is solidified, or crystal clear like water when liquefied. RBD oil made from copra can be just as clear and white. You often can't tell the difference between them just by looking. The way to distinguish between them is by the smell and taste. RBD oils are bland. Virgin oils have a mild coconut flavor and aroma.

Some low quality copra oils are marketed as virgin or unrefined coconut oils. They often taste terrible. They have undergone less processing than most RBD oils. This doesn't mean they are more natural than refined copra oil (RBD); they are actually inferior quality RBD oils. These oils have a strong smell and taste and are slightly discolored. When coconut is dried in the open air, the copra becomes contaminated with bacteria and mold. If the oil is not completely refined, bleached, and deodorized, it will have a yellowish or gray color, the result of residue from the mold and other impurities. This residue is considered harmless because the heat used in the processing has rendered it sterile. You can tell the difference between these oils and true virgin coconut oil by the color. Because these oils contain a higher level of impurities than other coconut oils, they have a relatively short shelf life, about six months. This type of oil is used mostly in the making of soaps and cosmetics though they are often sold as cooking oil in Asian markets. These oils are less expensive to produce than virgin coconut oil and so are sold at a fraction of the cost. One of the signs of inferior quality oil is the price. These oils sell for half the price of good virgin coconut oils. I don't recommend them because they taste horrible and contain too many contaminants. Even RBD oil is better. The coconut oil you use, whether it be virgin or RBD, should be colorless, not yellow.

Regardless of the method of processing, all coconut oils contain essentially the same amount of health promoting medium-chain fatty acids. These fatty acids are very resistant to heat and, unlike polyunsaturated oils, are not harmed in processing, even when high temperatures are used. For this reason, RBD coconut oil is still considered a healthy oil. You generally won't find the term RBD mentioned on labels, however, the only way you can tell is by the clear color and the lack of any taste or smell. Many people prefer this type of oil for all-purpose cooking and body care needs because it doesn't affect the flavor of foods or leave an odor when used on the skin.

Personally, I prefer the mild flavor and aroma of virgin coconut oil. It can be used to cook any type of food. Mild flavored foods such as eggs may taste a little like coconut, but most foods with a moderate flavor will completely mask the coconut. For some foods the coconut enhances the flavor. The biggest drawback to virgin coconut oils is that they are more expensive.

You will find a wide degree of difference in the taste of some of the oils. Some people don't like the taste of coconut or don't like it combined in all their foods. Some brands have a very strong flavor. The flavor isn't from the coconut but from impurities. Highly processed tasteless oil would be preferable. I recommend that you try several different brands and use the ones that taste the best to you. If you like the taste of an oil, you are more likely to use it.

Characteristics of Coconut Oil

Coconut oil, being highly saturated, is very stable and extraordinarily resistant to oxidation. When oils oxidize, they become rancid and form toxic free radicals. Coconut oil is so stable that when heated, it is 12 times more resistant to oxidation than canola oil, 16 times more resistant than soybean oil, and 300 times more resistant than flaxseed oil. To equal the amount of oxidative damage that occurs in flaxseed oil in just 30 minutes of heat processing, coconut oil would have to be subjected to the same conditions for 150 continuous hours—that's over six days! Because coconut oil is so chemically stable, it is one of the best (safest) oils to use for cooking and has a long shelf life. If processed properly, it can be stored for two or three years or more without going rancid. I've heard of oil that was as much as 15 years old without it becoming rancid. When used in cooking, it can be heated and reheated without producing damaging free radicals.

Although coconut oil is stable when heated, it has a moderate smoking point when used for frying. You need to keep the temperature under 350 degrees F (175 C). If you don't have a temperature gauge on your stove, you can tell when it goes over this point because the oil will begin to smoke. This temperature is moderately hot, and you can cook anything at this heat, even stir-fry vegetables. When used to grease pans or in baked goods, coconut oil can be cooked in the oven at higher temperatures because evaporation of water in the food keeps the temperature lower.

Because coconut oil is very stable, it does not need to be refrigerated. It will stay fresh for at least two or three years unrefrigerated. If kept in a cool place, it will last even longer. I buy mine by the gallon so that I always have an ample supply on hand.

An interesting characteristic about coconut oil that mystifies some users is coconut oil's high melting point. You can buy a bottle of liquid clear coconut oil in the store and take it home and the next day it has transformed into a hard, white solid. Some people might think it has gone rancid, but it hasn't. Coconut oil turns from a clear liquid into a hard, white solid at temperatures below 76 degrees F (24 C). This change from liquid to solid isn't strange or unusual; butter does the same thing. Pull a cube of butter out of the refrigerator and it is solid. Keep it on the countertop on a hot day and it melts, as they say, like butter. For this reason, coconut oil is sometimes referred to as coconut butter.

If you live in a warm climate, coconut stored in the cupboard or on the countertop will remain a liquid. In cooler climates it will harden. You can use it either way. To liquefy hardened coconut oil, simply immerse the container in hot water for a minute or two. It melts quickly. I like using hardened coconut oil because I prefer to scoop out the amount I need with a knife or spoon rather than pour it out of the bottle; it is less messy.

Coconut oil can be used for all of your cooking and meal preparation needs just as you would use other oils. The only real difference is with salad dressings. Pure, 100 percent coconut oil doesn't make a good salad dressing, not because it doesn't taste good, but because of its high melting point. When liquid coconut oil is poured onto a cold salad, it hardens. It's like eating a salad with butter poured on it. Some people do eat it this way, but most prefer not to. This problem is easily solved if you mix another oil, such as extra virgin olive oil, into the coconut oil. With a mixture of half and half, the oil will remain liquid on the salad.

HOW TO MAKE YOUR OWN COCONUT PRODUCTS FROM FRESH COCONUT

In some areas it may be hard to find good quality coconut products that are free from preservatives, sugar, and other food additives. Some people don't like to use canned products and prefer to make their own so they can have truly raw coconut milk and cream. You can make your own coconut products directly from fresh coconut. In this section I show you how.

Coconut Milk and Cream

Materials: 1 fresh coconut, a blender, hot water, wide mouth mason jar (or other glass jar), cheesecloth.

To make fresh coconut milk, you need to start with a good quality coconut that is free from mold and contamination. Drain the water and remove the meat from the shell. You may also peel the brown membrane from the meat if you like, although this step is not necessary. Cut the coconut into 1-inch chunks and put them into a blender. Add a little hot water. Hot water helps to extract the juice from the meat. Use just enough water for the coconut to blend evenly. Too much water will overly dilute the milk. Blend the water and coconut for a few minutes until the coconut is thoroughly chopped.

If you freeze the coconut chunks and thaw them out before you blend them, you will be able to extract a little more of the juice. Freezing softens the meat, because the water expands on freezing and breaks the cell structure, releasing more fluid. Freezing does not affect the taste or nutrient content but it does make the coconut noticeably softer after it has thawed.

Fold the cheesecloth in half and lay it over the mouth of the mason jar. Pour about a fourth of the mixture onto the cheesecloth. Wrap the cheesecloth around the ball of wet coconut and squeeze tightly to separate the liquid from the pulp. Drain the liquid into the mason jar. After you have squeezed out as much liquid as possible, discard the pulp and repeat the process with the remaining portion of the blender mixture.

The liquid you have in the mason jar is fresh, raw coconut milk. If you let the milk sit for a while, it will separate with a creamy layer on top. This is coconut cream. Mix the milk and cream together before using. This method of extraction yields about 1 to 1½ pints of thick milk. You can dilute the milk with a little water to increase the volume to 2 pints (1 quart) if you like. Fresh coconut milk spoils quickly so use it soon after it is made. In the refrigerator it will last for about 3 or 4 days.

If you want only the cream, simply scoop it off the top. The bottom portion that remains is a skim milk. The fat content of the skim milk is lower and its taste is very mild.

A much easier method of making coconut milk and cream is to use a juicer. Most juicers, however, don't do a good job of extracting the liquid from fresh coconut except for the Green Star juicer. It generates virtually no heat and thoroughly crushes and presses the coconut instead of cutting or shredding it like other juicers. The pulp you get is dry indicating maximum juice extraction. You will get more juice from the coconut with this juicer than with the blender method described above. No water is used in this process so what you get is pure coconut cream. No heat is involved so the coconut cream is raw, a plus for those people who prefer raw foods.

Many people who are unfamiliar with coconut milk are surprised to find that it is not sweet. Some commercially canned milk and cream have added sugar. If you make curries, chowders, or sauces with coconut milk, you don't want it to be sweet. Coconut milk is very versatile; like cow's milk it can be used in a variety of ways and in both sweet and non-sweet foods.

Coconut Milk Drink

Materials: same as above but reserve the coconut water.

Follow the directions above but replace the hot water with the coconut water removed from the coconut. You might have to add some additional water to mix evenly in the blender. Using the coconut water gives the milk a slightly sweeter coconutty flavor. I like to add a pinch of salt to enhance the flavor slightly.

This coconut milk is excellent for drinking by the glass or in combination with breakfast cereal or fruit.

Dried Shredded Coconut

Materials: Same as the coconut milk (above).

An easy way to make dried shredded coconut is to use the leftover pulp from the coconut milk. Before putting the coconut meat into the blender make sure to peel off the brown layer (testa) with a vegetable peeler.

After extracting the milk, evenly layer the pulp on a cookie sheet. Place in the oven at a very low setting, about 120-140 degrees F (50-60 C). You don't want to cook the pulp, only dry it to remove the moisture. If you have a food dehydrator, it works best. Keep the shredded coconut in the oven for a couple of hours or until it feels dry. Use this coconut in any recipe that calls for shredded coconut. Store in an airtight container.

The coconut pulp you get after making the milk can be used in recipes without being dried first, but because it has a fairly high moisture content, it spoils quickly. If you refrigerate the pulp and keep it in an airtight container, it will last for about three or four days. You can also freeze it for up to six months.

Virgin Coconut Oil

Materials: Same as the coconut milk (above) and a small saucepan.

Virgin coconut oil has been made by individuals for home use for thousands of years. Although several methods are currently used, the fermentation method is the most traditional. The method described here is a slightly modernized (easier) method of the fermentation process.

To make the oil, you need to start with fresh coconut milk. Make coconut milk according to the recipe above. Use hot water and not coconut water in the blender. As soon as the milk is made you need to let it rest or ferment uncovered in the glass jar for 24 to 48 hours. Fermentation occurs best at temperatures between 85 and 105 degrees F (30-40 C). If your room temperature is not this warm, put the oil in a slightly heated oven.

As the oil ferments, a layer of curd forms on top. The water settles to the bottom and a very thin layer of oil forms between the two. The top two layers contain the oil. The most difficult part of the process is removing these layers from the water. The easiest method is to put the jar into the refrigerator for a few hours to let the oil harden. The curd, which is saturated with oil, will also harden. After the oil/curd has solidified, remove it from the jar. Discard the water. Put the oil/curd in a small saucepan, and heat the pan to 140 to 180 degrees F (50-60 C) for about 12 hours. Heating drives off moisture still trapped in the oil and helps separate it from the curd. The lower the moisture, the better the quality of the oil.

Remove the pan from the heat and let cool. You will have oil and coconut solids (mostly protein) in the pan. You need to separate the solids from the oil. Put a couple of layers of cheesecloth over the top of a wide mouth glass jar. Pour the oil mixture onto the cheesecloth and let the oil drain into the jar. Make sure the temperature of the room is above 76 degrees F (24 C) so the oil doesn't solidify. Let the oil drain for a couple of hours. Squeeze out any remaining oil from the curd and discard. This method will yield about 3 or 4 tablespoons of virgin coconut oil depending on the size of the coconut. The oil you get from this method will have a pleasantly mild, nutty coconut aroma and taste.

CULTURED COCONUT

Most people are familiar with cultured milk such as yogurt and kefir. Fewer people are familiar with cultured coconut. Fermentation of dairy involves partial conversion of the sugar in the milk (lactose) to lactic acid. The acid is what gives yogurt its sour taste. Coconut water and milk can also be cultured using the same organisms that are found in dairy milk. The natural sugar in coconut water feeds bacteria in a similar process. Coconut milk does not ferment well because it contains very little sugar. However, adding coconut water or granulated sugar to coconut milk will cause it to ferment.

Coconut kefir is made using kefir starter or grains and coconut water. Coconut milk can be used if you use a mixture of half coconut water and half coconut milk. For best results use water from a green or young coconut. Water from young coconuts is sweeter, tastes better, and will make a better cultured product. But you can make coconut kefir from the water of mature coconuts if that is all you have available.

The process is very simple. All you need is a wide mouth quart mason jar, coconut water, and kefir starter or grains. Kefir starter is easy to use. Combine the kefir starter with the coconut water in the mason jar. Cover to keep out dust and insects. Let the jar sit at room temperature for a few days. The longer it ferments, the stronger the flavor. When the flavor is to your liking, it is ready to drink. To store, cover tightly and put it in the refrigerator. Refrigeration doesn't stop the fermentation but slows it down. Save some of the kefir you just made and use it as the starter for the next batch.

If you use kefir grains instead of starter, the process is basically the same. The only difference is that you must remove the grains and use them for the next batch. Kefir grains look similar to clusters of tapioca. If you use kefir starter, you can make about 6 or 7 batches before the flavor starts to change at which point you need to buy more starter. If you use kefir grains, you can continue the culture indefinitely with no change in the flavor.

Complete details will come with the kefir. Although the instructions will be for milk, simply use coconut water instead. To obtain kefir starter or grains, go to your local health food store or look up "kefir" on the Internet.

COCONUT SOAP AND CLEANSERS
Basic Coconut Soap (Hand Soap)

Coconut oil has been used in soap making for years. It makes the best quality, richest lathering soaps. Most commercial soaps on the market today are made with coconut oil as the main ingredient. Soaps made with coconut oil are naturally antibacterial because they contain medium-chain fatty acids that kill germs. A unique feature of soaps made primarily from coconut oil is their ability to create a rich lather in hard water, including seawater. Other soaps can't do this.

Soap can be made from any type of oil or combination of oils. Usually coconut oil is combined with one or more other oils because pure coconut oil soap is very strong. Adding other oils makes a milder soap. The recipe described below uses 100 percent coconut oil and makes excellent hand soap.

Homemade soap is easy to make. All that is required is oil, lye, and water. The difficulty in making soap is taking the proper precautions when using lye. Lye is very caustic and will cause severe burns if it comes in contact with the skin. When working with lye it is recommend that you wear rubber gloves, protective eyewear, and work in a well ventilated area. If you're careful, you don't need to worry.

All ingredients are based on weight so you will need a scale that measures ounces. A kitchen or letter scale is sufficient. You will need a non-metal, heatproof bowl or container for the lye solution. I like to use a 1-quart mason jar. The thermometer is used to regulate temperature. It you don't have a candy thermometer, you can do without it. Do not use anything made with aluminum, including the thermometer.

You need to prepare a mold to hold the soap. The mold can be made from wood, cardboard, or plastic. Line the mold with plastic wrap to make the soap easy to remove after it has hardened.

Materials needed:
Kitchen scale
1-quart mason jar
Stainless steel or Pyrex saucepan
Stainless steel or wooden spoon
Candy thermometer
Soap mold

Ingredients:
6 ounces water
2.6 ounces lye
16 ounces coconut oil

Lye is sold in hardware stores as a drain opener. You may also find it sold in some grocery stores, chemical supply houses, and on the Internet. You want 100 percent lye. Lewis Red Devil lye is the most common brand. Look for lye in the plumbing department of the hardware store. Lye comes in crystal form. Keep the lid on the container tightly closed. Do not get any moisture in the container. When combined with water lye can become explosive. Never put water into lye, always put lye into water. Follow all the precautions on the container.

It is important that you follow these directions closely to avoid accidents and to get a quality product. Weigh out each ingredient. The directions call for 2.6 ounces of lye. If your scale isn't that precise, that's okay. Get as close as you can, 1 or 2 tenths of an ounce won't make much difference, but half an ounce will.

Step 1
Put the water in the mason jar and pour in 2.6 ounces of lye. You need to be in a well-ventilated area. Be careful not to breathe the fumes or splash any

of the solution on your skin. The water will become very hot. Place it aside to cool. Keep the mixture out of the reach of children.

Step 2

Put the coconut oil into a saucepan and heat to between 100 and 130 degrees F (38-54 C). If you don't have a candy thermometer, you can judge temperature by touch. It should be very warm, yet not so hot that you can't put your finger into the oil.

Step 3

When the lye solution has cooled to between room temperature and 95 degrees (35 C)—warm but not hot—slowly pour the lye solution into the oil, stirring constantly.

Step 4

The soap solution will be clear at first. As it cools it will slowly thicken and become white. You want it to become as thick as a milkshake which may take a couple of hours. You don't need to stir constantly the entire time, but check it often and stir frequently to prevent it from developing lumps. Keep the solution in a warm location.

Step 5

Take a spoonful of the soap solution and drizzle it back on top of the rest of the solution. If it piles on the surface without sinking, it is ready to be poured into the mold. Keep in the mold for 24 to 48 hours or until hard.

Step 6

The soap should be hard but not rock solid. At this stage you can still cut it fairly easily. Cut it into bars and remove from the mold. Allow the soap to cure for at least two weeks before using. If the soap is too soft after two weeks, let it cure until it hardens. To test if the soap is ready, wash your hands with it. If your hands become slimy and the soap won't come off, it's not done curing. Rinse your hands with vinegar and let the soap age a couple of more weeks.

This recipe makes an odorless hand soap. If you would like to give the soap a fragrance, you can mix in a little essential oil just before pouring the soap into the mold. Essential oils are extracts distilled from the fragrant portions of plants. They are called *essential* oils because they are the aromatic *essences* of the plants or flowers. The fragrance of some essential oils vanishes when mixed in the lye soap solution. If you use too much, the essential oils may alter the soap making process by accelerating the reaction and generating excessive heat. This can affect the outcome of the final product. If you use essential oils you should limit them to about 40 drops per batch. Some essential oils that don't affect the soap making process and are good to use are rose, lavender, eucalyptus, sandalwood, and clove.

Coconut Milk Bath Soap

Soap made with coconut milk is milder than the hand soap described above and makes good bath soap. Unlike pure coconut oil, coconut milk contains protein, which in my opinion makes a better soap. To make this soap you will need all the ingredients listed above plus the following:

2 tablespoons vegetable glycerin
20 to 40 drops essential oil (fragrance)
1 cup coconut milk

Follow the steps above for making the hand soap. Mix the glycerin into the coconut oil before pouring in the lye solution. The glycerin acts as an emollient, making the soap gentler on the skin. Mix the essential oil and coconut milk into the soap solution as it is thickening and almost ready to be poured into the mold. Adding the coconut milk will soften the soap solution, so allow it to thicken up a bit more before pouring it into the mold. Cure as described above.

Coconut Milk Shampoo

You can make your own rich lathering shampoo using any of the soap recipes described in this chapter. The recipe is essentially the same regardless of the type of soap you use. I prefer the Coconut Milk Bath Soap.

Take a bar of the Coconut Milk Bath Soap and with a knife or vegetable shredder shave off 1½ cups of soap flakes (loosely packed). Heat 1½ cups of water to a boil. Reduce heat to a very low setting. Add the soap flakes and let sit, stirring occasionally, until dissolved. Remove from heat and stir in ¼ cup of vegetable glycerin. Let cool. You may add a few drops of fragrance of your choice such as lavender or lemon oil. Use just enough to give the shampoo a slight aroma. Pour into a plastic squeeze bottle. The shampoo will be watery. If you want a thicker or thinner shampoo, adjust the amount of soap flakes you use, but don't use too much or the shampoo will turn into solid soap.

Coconut Palm Soap

A good all-purpose hand and body soap can be made from a combination of coconut and palm oils. Follow the directions described above for the Basic Coconut Soap but reduce the coconut oil to 8 ounces and add 8 ounces of palm oil. Decrease the amount of lye you use to 2.2 ounces. Everything else is the same.

You can make other soaps using different types of oils including olive oil. Follow the instructions for the Coconut Palm Soap and substitute olive or another oil for the palm oil. Do not change the amount of coconut oil. At least half of the oil you use needs to be coconut oil.

Degreasing Agent and Makeup Remover

Have you ever had your hands caked in grease and dirt or paint and tried to wash it off using ordinary hand soap? You can scrub until your skin is raw and still not remove it all. Grease, motor oil, oil-based paints, printing ink, varnish, and other oil-based products can be a nightmare to remove. The only things that seem to work are expensive anti-grease hand detergents and lava soap, which contains crushed rock and acts like sandpaper. There is another option: coconut oil—not coconut oil soap, just ordinary coconut oil. Coconut oil is an incredible degreasing agent. It cuts through grease like a hot knife cuts through butter. No more scrubbing for what seems like hours trying to get your hands clean. Take a teaspoon or so and work it over your hands as if you were washing your hands in the oil. The grease will dissolve and practically melt off your hands. After the grease becomes liquefied, wipe it off with a paper towel. Remove the remaining oil by washing your hands with ordinary soap and water. Your hands will be clean and spotless. It's that easy. If you want a little more scrubbing power, you can add a small amount of corn meal to the oil. This gives the oil some teeth to dig out imbedded grime.

Coconut oil makes an excellent natural makeup and mascara remover. No need to use petroleum-based mineral oils or expensive makeup removers. Just dab a little coconut oil on your hands and rub it onto your face. Wipe off the excess oil and makeup with a paper tissue and wash your face with bath soap. You face will look fresh and clean. You may want to apply a thin layer of coconut oil after washing with soap and water to moisturize and soften the skin.

COCONUT DETOX
Coconut Water Fast

Coconut can be useful as an aid in detoxification to cleanse toxins out of the body and accelerate the healing process. Fasting is the oldest therapeutic treatment known to man. It is mentioned in the Bible and in medical texts of ancient Egypt and Greece. Hippocrates, the father of Western medicine, was a proponent of fasting as a means of achieving better health.

Fasting relieves the body of the burden of digesting and eliminating food so it can focus on healing and cleansing. During this time toxins are removed and the healing process is accelerated. Water fasts were common in ages past and are still used today. With this type of fast a person would consume nothing but water for several days. Fasts would last anywhere from one to 30 days or more. Many health clinics, especially in the early 20th century, relied on water fasting to cure chronically ill patients. These clinics achieved a great deal of success helping patients overcome numerable health problems ranging from asthma and allergies to kidney disease and cancer.

Juice fasting has now become the most popular form of therapeutic fasting. In fasting clinics it was found that using vegetable and fruit juices produced quicker results than water alone. The reason is that water provides no nutritional support. The body must rely on stored nutrients to satisfy its needs. Many people are nutritionally bankrupt to begin with. When the body's nutrient stores become depleted the healing process slows down. With juice fasting the patient is provided with a continual source of vitamins and minerals. Consequently, healing progresses at a faster rate. Another advantage is that the juice provides a small amount of energy that gives the body a boost. On a water fast you become very tired and lethargic, which makes you want to do as little as possible. Juices provide enough energy to carry on normal daily activities.

The juice of the coconut (coconut water) can also be used in fasting. In the early part of the 20th century, before there were antibiotics and other drugs, fasting was a popular method of treatment in health clinics. Physicians who used coconut water achieved good results. In the book *Super Health Thru Organic Super Food,* published in 1958, Dr. Raymond Bernard tells of a new Jersey City physician who achieved remarkable results with an exclusive coconut water regimen. He told of a case of a woman with advanced tuberculosis who was given up to die but regained her health after living on coconut water for six months. In another case an infant, unable to take milk or any other nourishment, was fed on coconut water for six months and thrived wonderfully, regaining its health. "This is understandable," says Dr. Bernard, "since coconut water provides a balanced form of nourishment, containing coconut proteins, fats, carbohydrates, minerals and vitamins, all in solution in the purest distilled water. Also it contains trace minerals which the coconut derives from the sea, and which most other foods lack. When liberal amounts of coconut water are taken, not only does one remain well nourished, without having to experience the disagreeable symptoms of a complete fast, involving extreme loss of weight and strength, but can continue one's normal life and activities."

Coconut water is very cleansing and alkalizing. Water from young or immature coconuts is preferred. But the water of a mature coconut, which is the type you get from coconuts sold in grocery stores outside the tropics, is usable too. Coconut water is now packaged and sold in containers. For fasting I would recommend you use *fresh* coconut water directly from the coconut, because it has not been heat treated or altered in any way. For the Coconut Water Fast, the only thing you consume is coconut water, plain (filtered) water and, if you like, fresh coconut meat. That's it. You may also drink the sugarless lemonade described on page 197. Try it for three days. You can do it for 7 days or longer if you feel up to it. You don't want to drink exclusively coconut water as it has a diuretic effect and you would be in the bathroom all day long. It also has a high amount of sugar that could feed candida, which is a problem with using sweet juices in fasting.

One of the major problems I have seen with juice fasting is that many people tend to use juices made from carrots and fruit. These juices taste good because they contain a high amount of sugar. The sugar feeds candida and has a negative impact on blood sugar, both of which can hamper healing. Better results are obtained using juices with a minimal amount of sugar. This is why vegetable juices are superior to fruit juices for cleansing and healing.

Coconut Oil Detox

This is a very powerful cleaning program and is ideal for correcting all types of digestive problems. This cleanse aids the body in rebalancing the environment within the intestines and healing damaged tissues. Systemic candida infections (candidiasis), inflammatory bowel diseases, leaky gut syndrome, and other conditions involving the digestive system are notoriously difficult to treat using conventional and even alternative approaches. Treatments last for months and may not be completely successful despite strict adherence to the various programs.

In this program you can drink as much filtered water as you like. In fact, you are encouraged to drink plenty of water. In addition to the water, you will consume coconut oil as part of a detoxifying beverage. The Coconut Oil Detox is the most effective method I have seen to rebalance the digestive system and get it functioning normally again. The detox consists of a beverage that is consumed at various times of the day. It is far superior to a simple water fast or even a juice fast. Juice fasts have one major drawback: they contain a lot of sugar. If you are trying to fight a systemic candida infection or an overgrowth of unfriendly bacteria, you don't want to keep feeding these microbes sugar, which they thrive on. Many people have gone on juice fasts hoping to overcome candida infections and improve intestinal function to find only minor relief. The sugar in most juices, even vegetable juices, keeps feeding unfriendly microbes. The Coconut Oil Detox provides very little sugar for these troublemakers to eat. So you essentially starve them to death. Coupled with coconut oil's germ-killing properties, the environment in the intestinal tract becomes extremely inhospitable to microscopic troublemakers. These unfriendly microbes naturally die off, leaving room for the good guys to repopulate and regain control of their natural habitat.

While on this fasting program don't be surprised if you expel from your bowels some awful looking stuff. Your body is cleansing all types of noxious debris. I have seen broken masses of fungus (candida rhizoids) that together would equal the size of a man's fist expelled during a fast. So don't be shocked at what you might find.

One of the benefits of juice fasting is that the small amount of calories it provides gives you enough energy to function throughout the day without becoming overly fatigued. With coconut oil you have a better source of calories in the form of MCFAs. These fats do not feed unfriendly microbes, but they do feed the cells and tissues in the intestinal wall and thus promote healing. They also boost our energy level so that we can function normally without any additional food or source of calories. During this cleanse you consume a large amount of coconut oil, far more than you would ever think of eating normally. Don't worry about eating so much oil; it won't do you any harm and will accelerate the rate of healing.

You will also be consuming a source of soluble fiber. I recommend ground or powdered psyllium husk. Psyllium husk serves several important purposes. First, it provides bulk to help you feel full and ease hunger. Second, it provides a source of food for your friendly gut bacteria to feed on and encourage their growth. Third, the bacteria that feed on this fiber produce SCFAs, which are used as food to nourish the cells lining your intestines. SCFAs provide these cells with the energy they need to function properly and to instigate healing and repair. Fourth, it helps prevent nausea and diarrhea that often accompanies the consumption of large quantities of coconut oil. When fats are consumed, the glycerol portion of the triglycerides is separated from the fatty acids. A large amounts of glycerol causes water to be drawn into the intestines, which leads to the nausea and loose stools some people experience when they eat a lot of fat or oil. Soluble dietary fiber, such as psyllium husk, absorbs this excess fluid preventing these side effects. Fifth, it acts as a colon cleanser, allowing you to have somewhat regular bowel movements to clear out the garbage in your colon.

The detox beverage includes a small amount of coconut water and unrefined sea salt, both of which provide important electrolytes that quickly become depleted during detoxification and water fasting. Coconut water provides the base into which the coconut oil and other ingredients are combined. The mild sweetness of the coconut water makes the drink a little more palatable. The small amount of natural sugar in the coconut water is completely metabolized into energy without providing any food for your gut microbes. Coconut water also contains several phytonutrients that are health-promoting and will aid in the detoxification process. You can use the water from a fresh coconut (preferred) or from any of the commercially packaged coconut water products available in most stores. If you use a commercial product read the ingredient label and make sure it contains only coconut water and no additives.

To make the Coconut Oil Detox beverage you need the following ingredients:

2 tablespoons coconut oil
½ cup coconut water
1-2 teaspoons psyllium husk
Pinch of sea salt

The beverage needs to be slightly warm to allow the coconut oil to blend in. Heat the coconut oil until it is liquid and very warm or slightly hot and then pour it into a small glass. Stir in the coconut water, psyllium husk, and salt. Use a large enough two-finger pinch of salt to make the beverage mildly salty without being overpowering. Set it aside and let it rest for about 5 minutes; this allows the psyllium husk to absorb some of the water and soften. If you drank the mixture immediately the psyllium husk would feel grainy in your mouth and throat. Once it has absorbed some of the liquid, it becomes soft and the beverage thickens with a slight gelatinous texture. Stir it up and drink it all. Follow with a glass of water.

This entire beverage should be consumed between 3 to 5 times during the day. Most people, especially if this is their first time doing the detox, limit it to 3 times daily. Start in the morning and consume it every 2 to 3 hours or so. Make it fresh each time as the beverage becomes more gelatinous as it sits, making it a little harder to consume. For some people, eating coconut oil in the evening gives them so much energy it makes it difficult for them to fall asleep at night. I recommend that you avoid drinking this beverage within three or four hours before going to bed. Make sure you drink plenty of water during the day.

The Coconut Oil Detox beverage doesn't taste too bad. Some people like it. Others, however, have a hard time swallowing it. If you are one of these, there is an aid you can use to help with the taste and texture. This method involves mixing a little plain yogurt into the beverage. The beverage becomes almost like a soft pudding. The yogurt you use must be unflavored, unsweetened, and preferably organic with live cultures. The cultures are an added bonus because they help repopulate the intestinal tract with friendly bacteria. It is very important that you do not use sweetened yogurt, as the sugar feeds candida. Prepare the Coconut Oil Detox beverage as described above. Vigorously stir in 2 to 4 tablespoons of unsweetened yogurt blending it well with the other ingredients. Let it sit for a few more minutes to thicken, stir and drink or eat with a spoon.

During the cleanse you consume only filtered water and the Coconut Oil Detox beverage—nothing else except plain yogurt if you choose that method. You will feel a little hungry at first but you will not starve or become malnourished. You could live on this diet for months without harm. So there is no need to worry about not getting enough to eat. After the first day your hunger will fade and you won't feel like eating. If foods are placed in front of you, you'll have desires to eat them but as long as food is out of sight you will not feel the need to eat.

The Coconut Oil Detox is an ideal method to clean out and rebalance the digestive tract. It is very cleansing and will help with virtually any gut related health problem. The cleanse can be done for 3 or 7 days or even longer. For longer periods of time, however, I recommend you seek the guidance of someone experienced in fasting to help you along the way. Shorter fasts of 7 days or less you can do on your own. Most anyone can do a 3 day Coconut Oil Detox. If you have serious health problems you may want to check with your doctor before doing it longer. You may want or need to do *several 3 day cleanses*. The benefit of the longer fasts is that cleansing is quicker and after the first day or so hunger is greatly diminished so continued fasting becomes much easier.

Because most people who have health problems also have a poor diet, their nutritional status is low. They have few, if any, nutritional reserves. I recommend that before going on a fast, you take between 2 and 4 weeks to prepare. Take a multivitamin and mineral supplement daily. Focus on eating more fresh vegetables. Eat at least 8 servings of vegetables a day. Have at least one salad a day as your main meal. Add at least 1 and up to 3 tablespoons of coconut oil to your diet every day. Eliminate sweets, coffee, alcohol, white rice, white bread and flour products, and junk food. If you do this before the fast, you will get better results and have a much easier time.

If on the detox your stomach feels queasy, drink more water to help settle it. If after a few days you begin to experience low back pain, eat more salt and make sure you are consuming plenty of water. It is important that you get an adequate amount of salt during the fast because you are losing salt every day. One sign that you need a little more salt is if water begins to taste stale or dull rather than refreshing, as it should. Remember to use only unrefined sea salt and not regular table salt. You might also increase *slightly* the amount of coconut water used in making the detox beverage.

One of the things you may experience during the cleanse is a healing crisis (see page 176). This is one reason why on extended fasts it is beneficial to have the help of an experienced health care professional. The healing crisis can bring about some uncomfortable symptoms as a result of heavy cleansing. It is nothing to fear or worry about. It is a sign of improving health, and you should feel glad if it happens because it means you are getting healthier and will feel much better when the cleanse is over.

PARASITE PURGE

This process is based on traditional methods and has proven to be successful in expelling tapeworms and other intestinal parasites. The key to making this process work is eating an adequate amount of dried coconut. Dried coconut is more effective than fresh in cleansing out parasites. You need to eat about 2½ cups of dried desiccated or shredded coconut followed by a strong laxative. The combination of the coconut and laxative is very effective in flushing parasites out of the intestinal tract. Cloves can be added to kill the parasite eggs. It does little good to remove the parasites and leave the eggs, which will eventually develop into more parasites.

Since the Parasite Purge will loosen your bowels and cause you to visit the bathroom frequently for a few hours, you need to choose a day that will allow you to do this. You will start the purge the day before. If you choose Saturday as the day that you need to be near the bathroom, you will begin the purge Friday night or Friday afternoon. Saturday morning you will need to be close to a bathroom. By noon on Saturday you should be back to normal.

The first stage of the Parasite Purge is to eat 2½ cups of dried coconut. If you can eat this much at one time, have the meal in the evening. If it takes you two meals to down this much coconut, eat it for both lunch and dinner. If you need longer, eat it between meals or even for breakfast if you have to. After you begin eating the coconut, do *not* eat any other food! Drink plenty of water.

About two hours after your evening meal, mix 1 tablespoon of Epsom salt with ¾ cup of water. Drink this mixture. Epsom salt has an unpleasant taste. Using a straw will make it easier to get down. You may also add a little vitamin C powder or lemon juice to mask the taste somewhat. Drink the entire thing quickly. Follow with a full glass of water.

Wait about two hours. Before going to bed, drink another mixture of 1 tablespoon of Epsom salt with ¾ cup of water. Follow with a glass of water.

In the morning you will experience loose, runny stools and will need to empty your bowels a few times. If you have any parasites, you will see them floating in the toilet bowl. You can tell they are parasites because they may be alive and moving.

Eating 2½ cups of dried coconut is not easy for many people unaccustomed to using coconut in food preparation. Below are two recipes, one for Coconut Porridge and the other for Coconut Macaroons that provide a palatable means to eat the coconut. You can eat either one or use a combination of both to get your 2½ cups of dried coconut.

Coconut Porridge
1¾ cups water
1¼ cups dried finely grated coconut (unsweetened)
½ cup raisins or chopped prunes
1 tablespoon honey
½ teaspoon ground cloves
¼ teaspoon allspice (optional, added for flavor)
Salt to taste

Heat water in a saucepan until boiling. Add grated coconut, raisins, honey, cloves, allspice, and salt. Reduce heat and simmer for about 8 minutes or until raisins are very soft. Remove from heat. Serve warm topped with yogurt or coconut milk. You may also serve the porridge with fresh fruit. Goes well with sliced peaches, mangos, or pineapple. Drink with lots of water.

You will notice this recipe contains only 1¼ cups of coconut, one half the amount of coconut you need for the purge. You can double this recipe for the full amount. However, this recipe is usually more than enough to fill a person up at one sitting. You may need to make a second batch later to get all the coconut you need. Eat as much of the coconut as you can in one sitting. If you cannot get a full 2½ cups worth, prepare it again and eat it at the next meal or eat the Coconut Macaroons.

Coconut Macaroons
2 egg whites
Dash of salt
½ teaspoon almond or coconut extract
6 tablespoons coconut sugar
1¼ cups shredded or grated coconut

Beat egg whites, salt, and vanilla until soft peaks form. Gradually add sugar, beating until stiff. Fold in coconut. You may also add ½ teaspoon of ground cloves if you like, but the cloves are optional. Drop by rounded teaspoon onto a well-greased cookie sheet. Bake at 325 degrees F (165 C) for 20 minutes. Let cool about 1 minute; then while still hot remove cookies carefully from the pan. As the cookies cool, they tend to stick so it is easier to remove them while they are still hot. Makes about 1½ dozen.

You will need to eat about 3 dozen cookies to get the 2½ cups of coconut. These cookies are small and fairly light so eating this many isn't as difficult as it may seem. Combine the cookies with the Coconut Porridge over the course of the day to get the total amount of coconut you need. You don't have to use these recipes. Any recipe that includes a fair amount of coconut can be used. Besides shredded or grated coconut, you can also use coconut flour. Coconut flour is more concentrated than shredded coconut. You only need about 1¾ cups of coconut flour to get the same effect as 2½ cups of shredded coconut.

FORMULAS AND RECIPES

In this section you will find a number of formulas and recipes designed to aid in certain health issues. Most of these formulas and recipes use coconut milk or oil.

Coconut Cottage Cheese

This is a simple and tasty way to get a daily dose of coconut oil into the diet. You can adjust the amount of oil you use so that you can get two or more tablespoons at one time if needed.

1 to 3½ tablespoons coconut oil
1 cup cottage cheese
1 cup strawberries or peaches
¼ cup shredded coconut (optional)

Put melted coconut oil and cottage cheese in a blender or food processor. Blend until smooth. Pour into a bowl. Stir in shredded coconut (to increase fiber content) and fruit.

Coconut Spice Drink (Blood Sugar Control)

This is a tasty drink you can use to help control blood sugar levels. Both the cinnamon and coconut moderate blood sugar. This drink slows down the release of sugar into the bloodstream and prevents spikes in blood sugar.

1 cup coconut milk
¼ cup water
½ tablespoon cinnamon
⅛ teaspoon ground allspice or nutmeg

Combine the coconut milk and water in a small pan. Stir in cinnamon and ground cloves or nutmeg. Bring it to a simmer and heat for about 5 minutes to blend in spices. Cool and drink. Makes one 10-ounce serving.

Coconut Ginger Drink (Nausea and Indigestion)

This creamy beverage is good for relieving nausea, indigestion, and motion sickness.

½ cup water
1 teaspoon fresh ginger, thinly sliced
1 cup coconut milk
1 teaspoon honey

In small saucepan, heat water to boiling, add ginger, reduce heat and simmer for 10 minutes. Turn off heat, remove and discard ginger, and stir in coconut milk and honey. Serve warm.

Arthritis Ginger Tea

This tea is good for restoring health to joints affected by arthritis. Use as much ginger as you like. The more ginger, the better because it helps to reduce inflammation. Bring ½ cup of water to a boil. Cut the ginger into thin slices, put them into the hot water, and simmer for about 5 minutes. Remove the pan from the heat and discard the ginger. Stir into the hot water ¼ teaspoon of powdered turmeric and 1 tablespoon of unflavored gelatin. Add 1 tablespoon of coconut oil and continue to stir until the gelatin is dissolved. Add ½ to 1 cup of calcium enriched orange juice. Beverage should be consumed once or twice daily.

Health Tonic

This is a delicious tasting, all-purpose health tonic packed with vitamins and minerals that will give you the energy you need to start off your day. Although great for breakfast, it can provide you a nutritional boost any time of day. It's good served warm and tastes much like a light tomato soup. Goes well with coconut oil, making a convenient way of adding the oil into the diet. It's a healthy alternative to a morning cup of coffee.

1 cup fresh vegetable juice*
½ cup hot water
2 tablespoons coconut oil
¼ teaspoon onion powder
1 can (8 ounces) tomato sauce
1½ teaspoons fresh lemon juice
¼ teaspoon sea salt
Pepper to taste (optional)

Using a juicer, make 1 cup of vegetable juice. Use a mixture of different vegetables to get the best combination of nutrients. Vegetables that work well are carrots, beets, celery, chard, spinach, cilantro, bell pepper, and zucchini. Cruciferous vegetables such as cabbage, cauliflower, broccoli, turnips, and bok choy have a strong flavor. If you use any of them, use them sparingly.

Heat ½ cup water, coconut oil, and onion powder until hot, making sure the oil is completely melted. Stir together the hot water mixture, tomato sauce, vegetable juice, lemon juice, and add salt and pepper to taste. The beverage should be warm enough to keep the coconut oil melted. If the flavor of the tonic is too strong, dilute it with a little more water. Stir and enjoy. Makes two servings.

*If you don't own a juicer you can substitute water for the vegetable juice. Combine 1½ cups water, tomato sauce, and onion powder in a small saucepan. Heat until hot. Remove from heat and stir in lemon juice and coconut oil. Add salt and pepper to taste. Stir and enjoy.

Sore Throat Syrup

This is a traditional remedy used in Southeast Asia that reportedly works wonders for soothing a sore throat. The original recipe calls for coconut or palm sugar, which is made from the sap of the coconut blossom. If you don't have coconut sugar available, you may substitute sucanat (raw sugar), molasses, or honey.

1 tablespoon coconut sugar
⅛ teaspoon cracked peppercorns
1 teaspoon powdered turmeric or turmeric root
1 cup water
½ cup coconut milk

Combine the sugar, peppercorns, turmeric, and water in a saucepan. Bring to a boil and reduce heat and simmer until liquid is reduced by half. Remove from heat, strain, and add coconut milk. Take two tablespoons every hour or two.

Paul Sorse's Bowel Cleanser

This was one of Paul Sorse's favorite treats. He recommended it for those people who needed a little help with regularity.

1 cup dried or fresh apricots
1 cup dried pitted prunes
1 cup water
½ tablespoon fresh ginger, chopped
½ cup yam, cooked
1 cup coconut milk
2 tablespoons coconut sugar or honey

Soak dried fruit overnight in water. Steam or bake yam until soft and set aside to cool. Place fruit and ginger in a pot, adding just enough water to almost cover the fruit. Do not use too much water. Simmer until soft, about 30-40 minutes. Remove from heat and let cool for a few minutes. Put the fruit into a food processor or blender and add coconut milk, yam, and sucanat or honey and puree until you get the consistency of a thick smoothie or a pudding. Add more yams to thicken if needed. Serve warm. You can serve it like a pudding or use it as a topping on fresh cut fruit, pancakes, banana nut bread, oatmeal, etc.

Colon Cleansing Formula

This formula is for those people who have serious constipation problems. It will cause you to empty your bowels frequently as it flushes encrusted and putrefied waste from your system.

½ cup apple juice
2 tablespoons liquid chlorophyll
2 tablespoons aloe vera juice
1 tablespoon coconut fiber or coconut flour

Mix all ingredients together and drink. Follow with a full glass of water taken with 2 cascara sagrada capsules. Cascara sagrada is an herb that promotes movement of the bowels. It is non-habit forming and can be used safely every day for extended periods of time.

This drink should be taken every evening for 30 to 60 days. Thereafter, it can be taken every other day indefinitely. Taking it in the evening allows it to work during the night so you can relieve yourself in the morning and not be troubled for most of the rest of the day.

Cayenne Poultice

1 part cayenne pepper
1 part coconut oil

Heat coconut oil until hot. Mix cayenne pepper and hot coconut oil together to form a paste. Let cool. Apply to skin and keep in place with a bandage. During the day add more coconut oil if necessary to keep the poultice moist. Reapply every day. Used for healing wounds and to stop bleeding. Reputedly this is more effective than traditional herbal remedies such as comfrey and aloe.

Oregano Ointment

This ointment is made from a combination of coconut and oregano oils. Oregano is known best as a seasoning in pizzas and Italian foods. It's also an effective fungicide. Its antifungal properties are concentrated in the oil portion of the herb. Oregano oil is an essential oil sold in health food stores. Do not use the dietary supplement form because it is diluted with other oils. You want pure essential oregano oil. The essential oil of oregano is a very strong and will burn your skin on contact, so be careful. Use it only when diluted with coconut oil. The formula for this ointment is simple; all you need to do is mix the following:

1 part oregano oil
5 parts coconut oil

Apply the oil topically. It works for ringworm, jock itch, athlete's foot, toenail fungus, dandruff, diaper rash, ear fungus, and any other fungal related condition. Deep-seated toenail fungus is notoriously difficult to treat. Even with prescription medications it takes weeks if not months to heal. This ointment works miracles in a matter of days. It's an excellent solution to dandruff; just rub a little of the ointment in the hair and massage it into the scalp. For most fungal infections rub the oil into the infected area at least once a day. An easy way to apply the ointment is to use the end of a cotton swab soaked in the oil. If the skin is sensitive, the ointment may burn a little. That's okay. The aroma of oregano is strong but quickly fades so you don't need to worry about smelling like a pizza all day.

Peppermint Ointment

This ointment is good for relaxing sore or stressed muscles and reducing inflammation. Great for back pain caused by cramps or sore muscles. Use a liberal amount of the ointment and massage it deep into the affected area. Work the oil into the skin so that it penetrates into the tissues. Make sure you use essential peppermint oil and not peppermint extract.

1 part peppermint oil
5 parts coconut oil

Clove Ointment

This ointment is good for bacterial infections. Use topically on the skin or gums. Good for fighting gum disease and dental plaque. Apply the ointment with a cotton swab. Clove oil is sold in the essential oils area of your health food store.

1 part clove oil
10 parts coconut oil

Bone, Joint, and Cartilage Ointment

The basic herbal formula for this ointment has been used by herbalists for many years and has produced excellent results. I've reformulated it using coconut oil, and the results have been remarkable. The combination of healing herbs plus the health benefits of coconut oil make a powerful healing combination. This ointment is intended for external use, but a tea can be made from the herbs for internal use if desired.

This ointment is useful for any injury to skin, bones, cartilage, muscles, or tendons. Good for sprains, pulled muscles, bone spurs, varicose veins, skin eruptions, burns, cuts—just about any bone or soft tissue problem.

I've had good results with this ointment. My wife developed a stress injury in her wrist that became chronic and very painful. The pain was so intense she had difficulty using her arm and could not lift anything that weighed more than a couple of pounds. She tried every remedy she could find, both conventional and traditional—cortisone shots, ultrasound treatment, wearing a flexible cast, massage, acupuncture, etc.—nothing seemed to help. Pain and weakness persisted for five years. One day she slipped on an icy driveway and fell on the wrist. The pain was excruciating. Her arm was almost completely incapacitated. Three weeks later the arm was still stiff and swollen. In order to help her I took the original formula for this herbal remedy and modified it using coconut oil. I wrapped her arm and hand in the ointment and she wore it to bed. The next day we took off the bandage and were amazed at the results. The swelling had completely disappeared and she was able to bend and move her wrist more than she had been able to for weeks. We continued to apply the ointment and bandages every night and saw continual improvement.

Inspired by her success, I tried it myself. Eight months previously I had dislocated one of my fingers. At first I thought it was just a sprain because I was able to move the finger even though the effort was very painful. I tried several commercial ointments and salves without success. After a few weeks with no sign of improvement, I had a chiropractor take a look at it. He took hold of my finger and gave it a sharp yank and a twist and popped it back into place. I let loose with a scream that frightened everyone in the waiting room. It did help because I was able to use the finger again to some extent, but pain and stiffness persisted for weeks. Impressed by the recent success of my wife, I soaked a large bandage in the Bone, Joint, and Cartilage Ointment and wrapped it around my finger. The next day when I removed the bandage the finger had noticeably improved. The finger healed quickly without problem.

The ingredients for the ointment are as follows:

6 parts White oak bark
6 parts Comfrey root
3 parts Marshmallow root
3 parts Mullein leaf
3 parts Black walnut bark or leaves
3 parts Gravel root
2 parts Wormwood
1 part Lobelia
1 part Skullcap
Coconut oil

Place the herbs in a glass or stainless steel container. Add just enough melted coconut oil to completely cover all the herbs. The level of the oil should rise no more than ¼ inch above the herbs. To extract the healing essential oils and phytochemicals out of the herbs, place the container in the oven at 180 degrees F (82 C) for 4 hours.

Remove the pan and let cool. Strain the oil into another container. Put the herbs back in the original container and again fill it with melted coconut oil until all the herbs are just barely covered. Heat the second batch for 4 hours just as before and strain the oil. You can even do a third batch to pull out the remaining essential oils.

The ointment is ready to use. Because coconut oil acts as an antioxidant, the ointment will last for several months. You may store it in the refrigerator if you like.

Apply the ointment liberally to the affected area and massage it in. If the area is too tender to be massaged, soak it in warm ointment for 5 or 10 minutes and then wrap it in a bandage. If the affected area is large, you may use cotton strips to bandage the area. You should apply enough ointment to soak the bandage. To keep the oil from becoming messy and prevent it from getting on clothes and sheets, wrap plastic around the bandaged area. Put the bandage on in the evening and wear it throughout the night, every night, until the condition has healed.

For severe cases you can also attack the problem internally by making a cup of tea using the herbs in this formula and drink it three times a day. Use one teaspoon of the combined herbs without the oil. Pour boiling water over the herbs and let steep for about five minutes or until cool. Do not cook the herbs in the water. Add the hot water to the herbs. Strain out the herbs and drink the tea. You may add a tablespoon of coconut oil to the tea if you like. Drink the tea and apply the ointment for maximum results. For most conditions, however, the ointment alone is enough.

Chapter 9

REMEDIES:
AN A TO Z REFERENCE

In this chapter many health problems are listed for which coconut has proven to be beneficial. This chapter does not contain every possible condition for which coconut could be helpful. Paul Sorse recommended that people experiment and try the oil for nearly anything. If it works, great; you've discovered something that brings relief. If it doesn't, no harm has been done because coconut is harmless. The only harm that may arise is for serious conditions where you choose not to seek professional help.

The information in this chapter is based on published medical literature as well as the research and experiences of Paul Sorse, the author, and numerous others who have used coconut for various health concerns. This information is not intended to replace a one-on-one relationship with a qualified healthcare professional and is not intended as medical advice. It is intended for educational purposes and to share knowledge about the useful properties of coconut. I encourage you to make your own health care decisions based upon your research and, when necessary, in partnership with a qualified healthcare professional.

Aches and Pains

Heat coconut oil so that it is very warm, but not hot enough to cause discomfort when applied to the skin. Massage the oil deeply into affected areas. Work the oil into the skin and muscles to stimulate circulation. Drink 8 or more ounces of coconut water and eat 3½ tablespoons of coconut oil a day. If pain persists, try massaging the area with Peppermint Ointment (page 205).

Acid Reflux

See Digestive Disorders.

Acne

Wash face with soap and water. Apply a thin layer of coconut oil and massage it into the skin. Do this every morning. Complexion may get worse at first as toxins are expelled from the skin, but will improve in a few weeks with continued application.

Age Spots

These are also called liver spots. They indicate free-radical damage in the skin. Rub coconut oil into the area daily and consume a maintenance dose of oil or other coconut products. Avoid processed vegetable oils, sunscreen lotion, and tobacco. Consume more fresh, raw fruits and vegetables. Age spots fade slowly so be patient.

AIDS/HIV

Consume therapeutic dose of coconut as indicated on page 169. Eat a healthy diet consisting primarily of fresh, raw fruits and vegetables with ample amounts of coconut meat and milk. See a qualified health care professional to guide you through the healing process.

Allergies

See Sinus Congestion and Autoimmune Disease.

Alzheimer's and Other Neurodegenerative Diseases

For the prevention of Alzheimer's and other neurodegenerative diseases take 2-3 tablespoons (30-44 ml) of coconut oil daily and eat a low-carb diet. For treatment purposes take at least 5 tablespoons (74 ml) of coconut oil daily with meals. Divide the dosage and take a portion with each of the three meals consumed during the day. For best results, combine the coconut oil supplementation with a very low-carbohydrate diet, limiting total carbohydrate intake to 30 grams per day or less. For more detailed information about preventing and treating neurodegenerative disorders see my book *Stop Alzheimer's Now! How to Prevent and Reverse Dementia, Parkinson's, ALS, Multiple Sclerosis, and Other Neurodegenerative Disorders.*

Arthritis and Stiff Joints

Massage affected areas with coconut oil twice a day. To help bring immediate relief from pain, massage the area with a combination of cayenne pepper and coconut oil.

Consume a cup of Arthritis Ginger Tea (page 202) three times a day. Get 1000 IU of vitamin D a day preferably from sunlight as described on pages 76-80, 500 to 800 mg of magnesium, 1000 mg vitamin C, and 100 mg grape seed extract. Avoid processed vegetable oils, sweets, and refined grains. Eat a high fiber diet rich in coconut meat, whole grains, beans, and fresh fruits and vegetables. Eat six to nine servings of fresh fruits and vegetables a day without overeating. Eat at least half of them raw. Replace sweets and refined and overly processed foods with produce. Eat fresh salads often with apple cider vinegar based salad dressings.

A toxic colon can have an affect on arthritis. A quick method of cleansing the colon and the entire digestive tract is the Coconut Oil Detox (page 195). For a more complete discussion on how to reverse arthritis see my book *The New Arthritis Cure.*

Asthma

Drink 2-3 quarts of water daily. Add 1 to 2 teaspoons of sea salt to diet. Rub coconut oil into chest, neck, shoulders, and back twice a day. Take a maintenance dose of coconut oil as described on page 168. Take 500 mg of magnesium and 500 mg of vitamin C daily.

Atherosclerosis

See Heart Disease.

Athlete's Foot

See Toenail and Foot Fungus.

Autoimmune Disease
(lupus, multiple sclerosis, fibromyalgia, allergies)

Consume the maintenance dose of coconut oil as described on page 168. Get 1000 IU of vitamin D a day, preferably from sunlight as described on pages 76 and 80. Take 500 to 800 mg of magnesium, 1000 mg vitamin C, and 100 mg grape seed extract. Consume the Coconut Ginger Drink or the Arthritis Ginger Tea (page 202) at least once or twice daily. Avoid processed vegetable oils, sweets, and refined grains. Eat a high fiber diet rich in coconut meat, whole grains, beans, and fresh fruits and vegetables. Eat six to nine servings of fresh fruits and vegetables a day without overeating. Eat at least half of them raw. Replace sweets and refined and overly processed foods with produce. Start a daily exercise program. Make the exercise vigorous enough to break a sweat.

Autoimmune disease can be greatly affected by a toxic colon. To cleanse the colon and entire digestive tract you may want to do the Coconut Oil Detox (page 195). It may take several 3 or 7 day cleanses or an extended cleanse to get permanent results.

Back Pain

Massage coconut oil deep into affected area and apply heat to relax muscles. If pain persists use Peppermint Ointment (page 205) in place of coconut oil. *See also* Osteoporosis.

Bacterial and Viral Illnesses

Most common bacterial and viral infections can be treated with over-the-counter remedies or dietary supplements. The main defense you have against these infections is your immune system. If you strengthen your immune system, it will be able to successfully fight off the infection. The approach here is to give your immune system the support it needs to do the job.

Drink plenty of water to keep the body hydrated and to wash out toxins. Eat sparingly and don't eat unless hungry. Get plenty of rest. If possible, go outside and get some sunshine. Dietary supplements you should consider taking include grapefruit seed extract, elderberry extract, and thymus extract. Follow directions on the bottles. Take 1000 mg of vitamin C, 1 capsule of cayenne pepper three times a day, and the therapeutic dose of coconut oil as described on page 169. Supplements should be taken with food and spread throughout the day.

If you are nauseous and can't eat anything, then don't. Try to drink some water. Coconut water is especially good because of the vitamins and minerals it contains. Rub coconut oil into your skin to get the benefits this way.

In some cases antibiotics may be necessary, but only when you have a serious bacterial infection. If you have a viral infection, avoid antibiotics. Antibiotics are worthless against viruses and may cause undesirable side effects. One of the side effects of antibiotic therapy is candida overgrowth. This problem can be partially avoided if coconut oil is taken with therapy. If your illness is causing serious discomfort or doesn't improve within a few days consult a healthcare professional for advice.

If the illness is affecting your sinuses or your breathing, you may try massaging the Peppermint Ointment (page 205) into the chest and neck.

Bad Breath

See Halitosis.

Bed Sores

Disinfect area with hydrogen peroxide or colloidal silver. Apply coconut oil bandage as described on page 164. Keep bandage moist and change every day until healed.

Bee Sting

See Insect Bites and Stings.

Bladder Infection
> *See* Urinary Tract Infection.

Blisters
> *See* Cuts and Wounds.

Blood Pressure
> *See* High Blood Pressure.

Bloody Nose
> *See* Nose Bleed.

Body and Foot Odor
Body odor is caused primarily by bacteria and fungus living on the skin. Ironically, bathing can make the situation worse. The surface of the skin should be slightly acidic to make it inhospitable to troublesome microorganisms. Soap and water removes this protective layer, leaving the body susceptible to colonization by organisms that promote body odor. Coconut oil can help restore the body's natural balance and protect you from odor-causing germs. If you have a mild problem, all you need to do is rub a little oil under the arms, on the feet, and anywhere else it may be needed. If your problem is more severe, you can get better protection if you combine coconut oil with an acid solution. After bathing you can quickly reestablish a protective acid layer by rinsing the body with a mild acid solution. You can make an odorless solution with water and vitamin C or citric acid powder. Mix 1 teaspoon of powder into 1 cup of water. After showering, turn off the water, and coat your body with this solution, making sure to get it under the arms and in the groin area. Get out of the shower and dry off. Apply a layer of coconut oil over the entire body, paying particular attention to the underarms and groin. Works wonders.

If body odor persists or if it is particularly strong, use Oregano Ointment (page 204). Many people are particularly troubled with smelly feet. This problem is often caused by fungus. Wash feet with soap and water, dry, and massage in a thin layer of Oregano Ointment making sure to get it into the cracks and folds. Repeat daily.

Boils
> *See* Cuts and Wounds.

Breastfeeding
The quality of a mother's breast milk is dependent on her diet. To enrich the milk with health promoting MCFAs, the mother should consume coconut products, especially coconut oil every day. The maintenance dose of 3½

tablespoons a day is adequate. This should be done before delivery as well as when nursing.

Bruises

To reduce swelling and pain, apply ice to the injured area as soon as possible. Keep the ice on for 15 minutes, and then allow a 15 minute break. Repeat several times. Gently apply a layer of coconut oil. Coconut oil can be applied 4 to 8 times a day or you can use a coconut oil bandage as described on page 164.

Burns

For minor burns immediately apply something cold such as a cool wet tea bag to the injury for about 10 minutes. Afterwards gently apply a layer of coconut oil. Reapply the oil every couple of hours or until the pain is gone. For more serious burns, use a coconut oil bandage as described on page 164. Continue to use the bandage until healing is complete. For deep or large burns see a healthcare professional for treatment.

Bursitis

See Arthritis and Stiff Joints.

Cancer

Avoid all vegetable oils, hydrogenated oils, and sugar, even natural sugars as they all depress immune system function. Consume the maintenance or therapeutic dose of coconut oil as described on pages 168 and 169. Massage coconut oil into skin daily especially over the area where cancer is present. Focus on eating fresh fruits and vegetables, mostly raw. Cut out all overly processed and refined foods, including packaged convenience foods. Eat lots of fresh green salads made with coconut oil/milk based dressings. Take thymus extract as per bottle directions and an antioxidant supplement that supplies vitamin A, vitamin E, zinc, and selenium. Take enough vitamin C to equal at least 1000 mg and 100 mg of grape seed extract. Take a capsule of cayenne pepper with each meal to improve circulation and increase oxygen delivery to the cells. Get 1000 IU of vitamin D preferably from sunlight as discussed on pages 76-80. See a health care professional to guide you through the healing process. To learn more about treating cancer naturally see my book *Ketone Therapy: The Ketogenic Cleanse and Anti-Aging Diet*.

Candida Infection (Candidiasis)

Avoid taking antibiotics if possible. Eliminate sugar and sweets of all types. Limit fruit intake. Sweeten foods using stevia. Eliminate all refined carbohydrates: white bread, white rice, etc. Consume a maintenance or therapeutic dose of coconut oil as described on pages 168 and 169. Eat a high fiber diet consisting of coconut meat, whole grains, beans, and fresh vegetables. Fiber is essential because it is converted into substances that help kill candida in the bowel. Eat yogurt or kefir daily. Take 1000 mg of vitamin C plus grapefruit seed extract and thymus extract as per bottle directions until symptoms improve. Get 20 to 30 minutes of direct full body sunlight each day. Start a regular exercise program. If a vaginal infection is also present, see Yeast Infection.

Systemic yeast infections can be very difficult to treat. The most powerful method for attacking this problem is the Coconut Oil Detox (page 195). You may need to do several 3 day cleanses or at least one 7 day cleanse to get permanent results.

Carpal Tunnel Syndrome

Drink 2 to 3 cups of Arthritis Ginger Tea (page 202) each day. Get the maintenance dose of coconut oil as explained on page 168. This can be done by drinking the tea. Take a multivitamin supplement that contains all the B vitamins, particularly B-6. In addition take 1000 mg of vitamin C and 500 mg of magnesium. Eliminate processed vegetable oils, sweets, coffee, and tobacco. Eat 6 to 9 servings of fresh fruits and vegetables a day without overeating. Massage warm coconut oil into affected area twice a day.

Cataracts

Take the *fresh* juice from a coconut and with an eyedropper apply several drops into each eye. Soak a washcloth in hot water. Wring out the water, lie down, and apply the warm wet washcloth over the eyes for about 10 minutes. Consume the maintenance dose of coconut oil as explained on page 168. Take 1000 mg of vitamin C and 50 to 100 mg of grape seed extract daily. Eat a diet consisting mostly of fresh fruits and vegetables. *See also* Eye Disorders.

Chapped Lips

See Dermatitis.

Chicken Pox

See Bacterial and Viral Illnesses.

Chronic Fatigue Syndrome (CFS)

The exact cause of CFS is unknown but it is generally believed to be caused by a chronic infection that the body is incapable of completely eradicating. Any number or combination of viruses, bacteria, fungi, or parasites can contribute to chronic fatigue. The most likely causes are the herpes virus, Epstein-Barr virus, candida, and giardia. Coconut oil can be beneficial because it can kill many of the organisms that may be involved, plus it increases energy and stimulates metabolism, which improve immune function. A basic approach to CFS would be to support the immune system to allow the body to rid itself of the problem. A helpful regimen is to take grapefruit seed extract, elderberry extract, and thymus extract. Follow directions on the bottles and continue until symptoms improve. On a continual basis take 1000 mg of vitamin C, a capsule of cayenne pepper, and the maintenance dose of coconut oil as described on page 168. Supplements should be taken with food and spread out though the day. Go outside and get some healing sunlight as described on pages 76-80. Eat a diet rich in whole foods with lots of fresh raw fruits and vegetables. Incorporate coconut meat and milk into the diet. Cultured coconut (page 188) or another source of friendly bacteria would also be helpful.

Cirrhosis
See Liver Disease.

Cold Hands and Feet
See Hypothyroidism.

Colds
Drink lots of water. Take 500 to 1000 mg of vitamin C, preferably with bioflavonoids, daily. Look for a supplement that includes both. Drink chamomile or peppermint tea with a tablespoon of coconut oil. Massage muscles on the back of the neck, shoulder, and chest thoroughly twice daily with coconut oil. *See also* Sinus Congestion.

Cold Sore
See Fever Blister.

Colon Cancer
See Colon Health.

Colon Health
(constipation, colon cancer, colitis, Crohn's disease, IBS)
Coconut meat and oil repair, rejuvenate, clean, and vitalize the digestive system. From mouth to rectum, coconut cleans and polishes, strengthens and feeds tissues. It helps to improve the tone of intestinal muscles and balances pH. Therefore, all problems associated with the colon can be aided by the consumption of both coconut meat and oil. The first step to good colon health is to keep the pipes clean and flowing smoothly. To accomplish this the diet should contain at least 20 to 35 grams of fiber. Coconut meat is an excellent source of dietary fiber. Other good sources are whole-grain bread, bran, brown rice, beans, fresh fruit (plums, apricots, apples), vegetables, and nuts. Your

diet should consist mostly of fresh fruits and vegetables. Drink 2-3 quarts of water daily. Add 1 to 2 teaspoons of unrefined sea salt. Cut down on caffeine and alcohol intake. Both can make the stool dry and hard. Avoid long-term use of laxatives. They can irritate the rectal veins. Get regular exercise. Exercise helps to move food along the digestive tract and tones muscles. Take 800 mg of magnesium, 1000 to 2000 mg of vitamin C, and a maintenance dose of coconut oil daily. Also get about 1000 IU of vitamin D daily, the best source of vitamin D is from sunlight as described on pages 76-80. Last but not least, eat cultured coconut (page 188) or unsweetened yogurt regularly to help establish and maintain a healthy intestinal environment.

To quickly reestablish a healthy intestinal environment and heal damaged and inflamed tissues in the digestive tract, the Coconut Oil Detox (page 195) is the best approach. It may require several 3 days cleanses or one or more 7 day cleanses to achieve desired results.

Constipation

Start breakfast with a papaya or papaya smoothie. Two hours later take 1 tablespoon of coconut oil. Consume at least 3 tablespoons of coconut oil a day. *See also* Colon Health.

Crohn's Disease

See Colon Health.

Cuts and Wounds

If possible, wash injury with soap and water first. Then apply a small amount of hydrogen peroxide or alcohol to disinfect it. To stop bleeding, sprinkle cayenne pepper into wound or use the Cayenne Poultice (page 204). This will stop the bleeding within seconds.

If the injury is minor you can rub a little coconut oil on and leave it alone or perhaps add an adhesive bandage. If the injury is deep, soak a bandage or gauze pad in coconut oil and secure it over the injury with tape or an elastic bandage. Keep the injury moist with coconut oil. Change dressing daily and monitor progress.

Dandruff

Apply coconut oil or Oregano Ointment (page 204) to the scalp. Massage it into the skin. Use just enough oil to cover the skin, not drench your hair. Let the oil soak in for 10-30 minutes, longer is better. Wash the oil out of the hair and dry. To moisturize your scalp, rub a few drops of coconut oil between your hands and brush it into hair and scalp. Repeat every day or two.

Dehydration

Coconut water makes an excellent beverage to rehydrate the body. It contains sugars and electrolytes that quickly replenish needed nutrients. Water from young or immature coconuts is superior in taste and quality to that from mature coconuts but either will work. Limit consumption to about 16 ounces at any one time. Drinking too much all at once can loosen the bowels. Drink lots of plain water as well.

Dental Cavities

See Gum Disease and Tooth Decay.

Dermatitis

Massage warm coconut oil deep into affected area. Repeat 4 to 8 times a day until condition improves. For conditions that don't respond quickly you may need to use an oil soaked bandage as described on page 164. Daily exposure to 15 to 20 minutes of direct sunlight is also helpful.

Diabetes

Eliminate sweets, refined carbohydrates, and processed vegetable oils from your diet. Eat a high fiber diet that includes coconut meat, whole grains, beans, and plenty of fresh raw vegetables. Use coconut oil for all cooking purposes. Consume maintenance dose of coconut oil as described on page 168. Take a multivitamin supplement that supplies at least 50 mcg of chromium, 50 mg zinc, 500 mg vitamin C, and 500 mg magnesium. Take 1 to 3 capsules of cayenne pepper with each meal to improve circulation. Start an exercise program and get 20 to 30 minutes of sunlight a day. See a healthcare professional to monitor progress. A complete program to reverse insulin resistance, the cause of type 2 diabetes, is available in my book *Stop Alzheimer's Now*. Anyone with type 2 diabetes would benefit greatly by following the program outlined in this book.

Diabetic Retinopathy

See Eye Disorders.

Diaper Rash

Diaper rash is an infection caused by candida in the stool. Candida loves warm, dark, moist environments, which is exactly what is found in a baby's messy diaper. To relieve this problem, change the infant's diaper immediately after each bowel movement. Wash the skin thoroughly with soap and water. Make sure the baby's skin is completely dry. You may want to let the baby go without a diaper for a while to expose the infected area to air and sunlight. Rub coconut oil onto the infected skin. Coconut oil makes an excellent baby lotion and should be used every time the diaper is changed.

Digestive Disorders

Drink 2-3 quarts of water daily. Most of this should be between meals. Avoid using processed vegetable oils because they are hard to digest. This is particularly true if you have difficulty digesting fats. Use primarily coconut oil in cooking and food preparation. If you have a difficult time digesting protein, eat fresh tropical fruits such as pineapple, passion fruit, kiwi, pawpaw, or papaya with your meals. These fruits contain protein digesting enzymes that will aid in breaking down meat. You may also take a digestive enzyme supplement if you prefer.

Cayenne pepper and vinegar also improve digestion. They stimulate gastric secretions, providing more enzymes to break down the food. A cup of vinegar tea just before eating is a good way to start the gastric juices flowing and preparing the digestive tract for the meal. Vinegar tea may sound awful but it is actually quite tasty. To make it, combine 2 teaspoons of apple cider or coconut vinegar and two teaspoons of honey to one cup of hot water. You can also use lemon juice and water with a little sweetening (I prefer coconut sugar). An easy way to take cayenne is in a capsule. This way you avoid the burn. If taken on an empty stomach it may cause a little uneasiness so I recommend you always take it with meals.

One of the major causes of indigestion and heartburn is constipation. Eat high fiber foods. Coconut meat and flour are excellent sources of dietary fiber. Coconut oil, coconut water, raisins, and prunes all help loosen the bowels. Vitamin C is also helpful. Start with 1000 mg every day. Large amounts of vitamin C (5000 mg or more) can cause diarrhea. You may want to add more to help move things along. There is no harm in taking this amount.

The Coconut Oil Detox on page 195 may also be of great benefit. *See also* Colon Health.

Dry and Cracked Skin

See Dermatitis.

Dry Nasal Passages

During the winter in cold dry climates, nasal passages can dry out causing itching, burning, and the formation of mucus crusts. Traditional treatment is a salt water spray. Using coconut oil in place of salt water gives far better results. Using your finger, put a dab of oil up each nostril then lie down and let the oil drain into the sinuses.

Ear Fungus

Most people have ear fungus to some degree. It is evident by itching, excessive earwax, white powder, or flaky skin inside the ear canal. Fill an eyedropper part way with hydrogen peroxide and inject several drops into the ear canal. Do this lying down on your side or back. Get up. Let it dry. Put half a pea-size amount of coconut oil on your finger and coat the inside of your ear (I use a cotton swab). Every couple of days coat the inside of your ear with a small amount of coconut oil.

Ear Infection

Crush a fresh clove of garlic and mix the juice with a little coconut oil. Fill an eyedropper with the oil and put several drops into the ear canal. To prevent the oil from simply running back out and to get it deep inside the ear canal, lie on your side when you do this. Remain on your side for a few minutes. Open and close your mouth and move your jaw around to help work the oil down the canal. Stuff a small piece of cotton into the ear to prevent the oil from leaking out. Keep the cotton in the ear for about 15 to 30 minutes. To attack the infection from the inside, eat at least 3½ tablespoons of coconut oil per day. If you suspect a punctured eardrum, do not use this method.

Ear Wax

Excessive earwax can impair hearing and create a breeding ground for fungus and bacteria. Lie down on your side or back. Using an eyedropper filled with warm coconut oil, put several drops into the ear canal. Move your jaw around to work the oil down into the canal. This will loosen the wax and allow it to move out on its own. Repeat as often as necessary.

Eczema

See Dermatitis.

Eye Disorders

Most common eye disorders, such as glaucoma, macular degeneration, and diabetic retinopathy, are associated with excessive free-radical damage and poor glucose control. A low-carb or ketogenic diet limits carbohydrate intake and stimulates the production and use of ketones that can greatly improve glucose control and even reverse some of the damage caused to the retina and optic nerve. For a complete discussion on how to use coconut oil and diet to treat degenerative eye disorders see my book *Stop Vision Loss Now*.

Fever Blister

Also known as a cold sore, a fever blister is caused by the herpes simplex virus and usually appears on the face, generally around the mouth. Take a lysine tablet and grind it into a powder. Add coconut oil and apply to the infected area as soon as you feel the blister start to form. Cover with micropore tape and keep it on overnight. Take a maintenance dose of coconut oil as described on page 168 and 500 mg of lysine 3 times daily for two weeks. Do not take lysine for more than three weeks as it could create an imbalance in other amino acids.

Fibromyalgia

Take a maintenance dose of coconut oil and a multivitamin and mineral supplement daily. Massage painful areas with coconut oil or Peppermint Ointment (page 205). Participate in light aerobic exercise, such as walking, every day. Get at least six to nine servings of fresh fruits and vegetables daily. Avoid processed vegetable oils and hydrogenated oils.

Cleansing the body of toxins and improving intestinal health may be of great benefit. The Coconut Oil Detox on page 195 gives details. *See also* Autoimmune Disease. A complete program for treating fibromyalgia and arthritis can be found in my book *The New Arthritis Cure: Eliminate Arthritis and Fibromyalgia Pain Permanently*.

Flu

See Bacterial and Viral Illnesses.

Food Poisoning

See Bacterial and Viral Illnesses.

Gallbladder Disease

Those who have gallbladder disease or have had their gallbladder removed should avoid using all other types of fats and oils. Use coconut oil exclusively in all cooking. Use as much as your body can tolerate. This will vary from individual to individual. Fat is important in the diet as it is necessary for the proper digestion and assimilation of many important nutrients. Without adequate fat in the diet, you can develop nutritional deficiencies. Many protective antioxidants are fat-soluble vitamins that require dietary fat for optimal absorption.

Gangrene

Take the maintenance dose of coconut oil daily and 1 to 3 capsules of cayenne pepper with each meal to increase circulation. Apply coconut oil or a Cayenne Poultice (page 204) on the affected area. Seek medical attention.

Gingivitis

See Gum Disease and Tooth Decay.

Gum Disease and Tooth Decay

Paul Sorse brushed his teeth every morning with coconut oil and his breath was always fresh. Coconut oil kills germs that cause bad breath, tooth decay, and gum disease. It cleans the mouth, keeping it healthy. Adding a small amount of baking soda helps to neutralize acids that eat away tooth enamel.

For fresh breath, clean teeth, and healthy gums, brush teeth daily using a mixture of baking soda and coconut oil. Also, a practice known as oil pulling is remarkably effective in whitening the teeth, freshening the breath, healing gum disease, and pulling out infection. Basically all you do rinse your mouth with 1-2 teaspoons of coconut oil daily, spit out the oil after several minutes. Don't swallow it. A complete explanation of oil pulling and how and why it works is found in my book *Oil Pulling Therapy*. If you have any dental issues, I highly recommend you read this book. It can save you a lot of time, money, and pain from going to the dentist.

Hair Conditioner

Massage 1 or 2 teaspoons of very warm coconut oil or coconut milk into the hair. If possible wrap the hair in a hot towel. Let the oil soak into the scalp and hair for at least 30 minutes, longer if possible. Shampoo hair. You may also apply the oil at night before going to bed. Put on a bath cap, go to bed, and wash it out in the morning. After shampooing, rub a few drops of coconut oil between your hands and brush into your hair. You don't want to use a lot of oil, just enough to give it a healthy shine. Coconut oil gives the hair body and luster and gets rid of dandruff.

Halitosis

See Gum Disease and Tooth Decay.

Heart Burn

See Digestive Disorders.

Heart Disease

Take the maintenance dose of coconut oil as described on page 168. Eliminate all processed vegetable and hydrogenated oils from the diet including all foods that contain them. Eat a high fiber diet with lots of coconut meat, whole grains, beans, and fresh vegetables. Avoid sugar and sweets. Take a multivitamin supplement with all B vitamins (thiamin, riboflavin, niacin, biotin, B-12, folic acid, etc.) with at least 100 mg B-6. Get 1000 IU of vitamin D preferably from sunlight as described on pages 76-80. Take 1000 mg vitamin C, 500 to 800 mg magnesium, 100 mg grape seed extract, and 60 mg CoQ10. Take 1 to 3 capsules of cayenne pepper with each meal to improve circulation. With the permission of your doctor, start an exercise program.

Hemorrhoids

First, disinfect the affected area with a cotton ball soaked in hydrogen peroxide. Gently massage coconut oil into area 4 to 6 times daily. Eat at least 3½ tablespoons of oil and take 1000 mg of vitamin C a day. Also helpful would be 100 mg of grape seed extract and a capsule of cayenne pepper with each meal. Continue until relief is achieved. Hemorrhoids often occur when there is constipation, so keep regular by eating high fiber foods. Coconut meat is an excellent source of dietary fiber. Other good sources are whole-grain bread, bran, brown rice, beans, fresh fruit (plums, apricots, apples), vegetables and nuts. Drink 2-3 quarts of water daily. Cut down on caffeine and alcohol. Both can make the stool dry and hard. Avoid long-term use of laxatives. They can irritate the rectal veins. Eat cultured coconut (page 188) or yogurt regularly. Exercise daily. Exercise helps to prevent constipation and also improves the strength of muscles supporting the rectal area. Finally, don't strain during bowel movements.

If hemorrhoids are severe, you might want to try using witch hazel because of its astringency. Saturate a cotton ball with distilled witch hazel, and apply to the hemorrhoid after each bowel movement and several times throughout the day to help shrink the swollen vein. Best results are achieved if you can leave the cotton pad on the affected are for 10 to 15 minutes if possible. Then apply a coat of coconut oil to speed healing. The Cayenne Poultice described on page 204 will also speed healing.

Hemorrhoids are often caused by an unhealthy digestive system. To correct this problem the Coconut Oil Detox (page 195) is recommended.

High Blood Pressure

Add more fresh fruits and vegetables into the diet—at least six to nine servings a day. Avoid all processed cooking oils. Use coconut oil for meal preparation and consume a maintenance does daily. Get 1000 IU of vitamin D a day preferably from sunlight as described on pages 76-80. Take 500 to 800 mg of magnesium. Take 1 or 2 capsules of cayenne pepper with each meal and a multivitamin supplement daily. Ten to 12 ounces of coconut water daily can help because it is a rich source of potassium

Hypertension

See High Blood Pressure.

Hypoglycemia

Many people report that after incorporating coconut oil into their diets, they no longer have sugar cravings or hypoglycemic symptoms. Consume the maintenance dose of coconut oil as explained on page 168. Snacking on fresh coconut meat throughout the day will also help keep hypoglycemic symptoms at bay.

Hypothyroidism

This is a complex problem that requires more discussion than we have space for here. Coconut oil can be of great benefit for many hypothyroid individuals. Some benefit more than others because many factors affect thyroid health. Coconut oil stimulates energy and metabolism and in this respect can be of benefit to all hypothyroid sufferers. With regular use it can stimulate metabolism enough in some people to permanently correct low thyroid function. Basically, you should consume the maintenance dose of coconut oil and avoid processed vegetable oils, raw cabbage family vegetables, and foods made from soybeans. Take 1 to 3 capsules of cayenne pepper with each meal to improve circulation and stimulate metabolism. For a more complete discussion on how to restore thyroid function see my book *The Coconut Ketogenic Diet.*

Immune System

Adequate sunlight, regular exercise, a diet rich in fresh fruits and vegetables, a positive mental attitude, adequate sleep, low stress levels, clean water, fresh air, and a maintenance dose of coconut oil all strengthen the immune system.

Indigestion

For acute cases of indigestion take 2 tablespoons of coconut oil. If needed take 1 tablespoon 6 hours later. *See also* Digestive Disorders.

Insect Bites and Stings

Massage coconut oil over the affected area. Warm oil penetrates deeper and gets the quickest results. Relieves stinging, itching, and inflammation. Apply two or three times a day.

Insect Repellent

Combining coconut oil with peppermint oil makes an effective natural insect repellent. See Peppermint Ointment on page 205. Rub it over all exposed skin.

Insomnia

Coconut oil helps regulate body functions that improve sleep. Consume the maintenance dose of coconut oil as given on page 168. Get 20 to 30 minutes of direct sunlight a day. Sunlight also helps regulate sleep. A cup of passionflower tea an hour before bedtime can encourage sleep. To make the tea, pour one cup of boiling water over one teaspoon of dried passionflower, cover, and let steep for 15 minutes. You may also add valerian root. Mix two parts valerian with one part passionflower, and make the tea as directed using one teaspoon of the herbal blend. Another thing you can do is take a relaxing Epsom salts bath just before bedtime. Add a cup of Epsom salts (magnesium sulfate) to a tub of hot water and soak for 20 minutes. Magnesium is an excellent muscle relaxant and sedative for the nervous system. Magnesium from the Epsom salts is absorbed through the skin during the bath has a relaxing effect on the body and mind.

Intestinal Parasites
Follow the instructions for the Parasite Purge on page 198. You need to allow a day and a half to complete the process.

Irritable Bowel Syndrome (IBS)
See Colon Health.

Itchy Ear
See Ear Fungus.

Itchy Skin
Coconut oil is excellent for soothing itchy or irritated skin. All you need to do is massage warm coconut oil into affected area. Repeat as often as necessary.

Jock Itch
See Skin Fungus.

Kidney Disorders
Eat a maintenance dose of coconut oil daily. Drink 16 ounces or more a day of coconut water. In addition, consume at least 6 eight-ounce glasses of pure water and 1 teaspoon of sea salt daily. Salt can be added to food or water. Take a capsule of cayenne pepper with each meal.

Kidney Stones
Drink 16 ounces or more a day of coconut water. In addition, consume at least 6 eight-ounce glasses of pure water and 1 teaspoon of sea salt daily. Salt can be added to food or water. Take a capsule of cayenne pepper with each meal.

Libido
Fresh young coconut water stimulates and strengthens reproductive functions especially in males. It is a natural alternative to Viagra. It is important that the water come from a green or immature coconut. The water in mature coconuts, the type normally found in grocery stores with the husk removed, is not as effective. The water must also be fresh. As soon as the coconut is opened, the water begins to lose this effect. Commercially produced coconut water that is sold in cans or Tetra Paks may have lost this effect.

Lice

Head lice are parasites that nest in the scalp and feed off the blood of the host. To get rid of them, start by removing as many lice as you can by combing your hair. To do this, massage a little coconut oil into the scalp and hair. Use just enough to barely coat the hair, not to make it oily. Comb through the hair with a fine-toothed comb. Pull the comb from the scalp to the ends of the hair. Rinse off any lice in the comb and continue. Comb through the hair at least twice. After combing, shampoo the hair thoroughly making sure to scrub behind the ears and at the back of the neck as this is where lice are most often found. Dry the hair. Apply a liberal amount of coconut oil or coconut milk and massage it deep into the scalp and hair. Keep the oil in the hair for as long as possible, at least 12 hours. Apply more oil or milk as necessary to keep scalp moist. If you do it at night, wear a shower cap to bed. Comb through the hair again and remove any lice you find. Most should be dead or gone by now. Shampoo the hair. Generally this regimen is enough to get rid of the lice. Repeat the process if necessary. For a stronger effect use Oregano Ointment (page 204) in place of coconut oil.

Liver Disorders

Liver problems such as hepatitis and cirrhosis can be helped by regular consumption of coconut oil. MCFAs in coconut oil protect the tissues of the liver from free-radical damage, which is one of the primary causes of liver injury. MCFAs also help fight infection. Follow the maintenance program on page 168. Dietary supplements containing an extract from milk thistle called silymarin can help rejuvenate and restore liver function. Take 1000 mg vitamin C daily. Avoid processed vegetable oil, hydrogenated oil, and alcohol.

Liver Spots

See Age Spots.

Low Stomach Acid

See Digestive Disorders.

Lupus

See Autoimmune Disease.

Macular Degeneration

See Eye Disorders.

Malnutrition

Use coconut oil in daily cooking and food preparation. Take a multiple vitamin and mineral supplement. Eat more fresh fruits, vegetables, and whole grains. Avoid processed convenience foods. Eat fresh coconut and coconut milk whenever possible and get the daily maintenance dose of coconut oil as described on page 168.

Moles

Moles can be removed using nothing more than coconut oil. Apply a bandage soaked in coconut oil to the mole (see detailed explanation on page 164). The bandage should remain moist with coconut oil. When it starts to dry out, add more oil. Keep the mole in constant contact with the bandage except to change it every day or so. Depending on the size of the mole, the process may take several weeks. If it takes longer than 6 days, remove the bandage one day to give the skin a rest. Continue in this manner six days on and one day off until the mole is gone.

Mononucleosis

See Bacterial and Viral Illnesses.

Mosquito Bite

See Insect Bites and Stings.

Multiple Sclerosis (MS)

See Autoimmune Disease.

Nausea

If you are able to keep anything in your stomach, take the Coconut Ginger Drink described on page 201.

Nose Bleed

Unless caused by an injury, bloody noses are often a product of the climate. Cold, dry air dehydrates nasal passages causing the mucous membranes to itch, burn, and crack. Irritation and mucus crusts encourage scratching. Softening and moistening the nasal passages will prevent dry cracked skin from developing and thus prevent bleeding. Coconut oil can easily accomplish this. Generously coat you finger with oil and rub it on the inside of your nostril. Lie down on your back and let the oil drain into your sinuses. To strengthen capillary integrity within the nasal passages, consume at least 500 mg of vitamin C and 25 mg of grape seed extract daily.

Coconut oil can stop bleeding as well. For mild nose bleeds, coat finger with a liberal amount of coconut oil and coat inside of the nostril. To prevent blood from going down the throat, sit down, lean forward and put your head down, leaving the mouth open for free breathing.

If bleeding is heavy, you can stop it almost immediately my using the Cayenne Poultice described on page 204. Coat the inside of the nostril with the cayenne Poultice as described above.

Obesity
See Weight Management.

Osteomalecia
See Osteoporosis.

Osteoporosis
Contrary to popular belief, osteoporosis is not simply a calcium deficiency disease. You can eat tons of calcium and still suffer from osteoporosis. Many factors contribute to osteoporosis. Take 800 mg magnesium and 1000 IU vitamin D daily. Avoid all processed vegetable oils with the exception of coconut oil. Use coconut oil or other saturated fats as your primary dietary fat. Eat some fat at each meal to improve mineral absorption. Vitamin D and saturated fat are necessary for proper calcium metabolism. The best source of vitamin D is from sunlight. Thirty minutes a day of full body summer exposure will supply the minimum amount needed. During the winter dietary vitamin D may be necessary. See discussion on pages 76 to 78. Avoid coffee, tea, soda, and sweets as they leach calcium from the bones. Get daily exercise to encourage bones to become stronger. A liquid trace mineral supplement is also recommended.

Parasites
See Intestinal Parasites.

Parkinson's Disease
See Alzheimer's and Other Neurodegenerative Disorders.

Poison Ivy or Oak
Apply a layer of coconut oil or Peppermint Ointment on affected area. Cover with a bandage. *See also* Dermatitis.

Prostate Enlargement
If you can get fresh green coconut water, drink one or two cups daily. Consume at least 3½ tablespoons of coconut oil a day. Massage coconut oil into the groin area daily. Take 200 IU of vitamin E, 200 mcg of selenium, and 50 mg zinc with copper, and a B complex multivitamin supplement. Eat at least 6 servings of fresh fruits and vegetables a day. Get daily exercise to improve circulation in the pelvic area. Avoid long periods of sitting. Get up and walk

around for a minute or two every half hour or so to stimulate circulation into the pelvic area.

Psoriasis

See Dermatitis.

Ringworm

See Skin Fungus.

Shingles

See Bacterial and Viral Infections.

Sinus Congestion

For relief of sinus congestion and respiratory problems, dip your finger into semi-hard coconut oil and fill each nostril. Lay down on your back with your head tipped back. Remain until the oil melts and goes down into sinuses (about 10 minutes). Be prepared to expel thick mucus. This will clear your sinuses and allow you to breathe easier. For a stronger effect use Peppermint Ointment (page 205). If the ointment is not solid, put it in the refrigerator for a few minutes. Also massage Peppermint Ointment into the neck and chest.

Skin Fungus
(athlete's foot, ringworm, jock itch, foot and nail fungus)

Massage coconut oil into infected area 3 to 6 times a day or use a coconut oil bandage as described on page 164. If possible, expose the infected skin to direct sunlight for 20 minutes a day (*see* Toenail and Foot Fungus). This procedure works very well and you should see new, healthy skin appearing within a week or so.

Skin and nail fungus is sometimes difficult to eliminate. If the above method doesn't completely remove the infection, repeat the procedure with Oregano Ointment.

Recurrent fungal infections are a sign of a systemic candida infection. The best way to treat this problem is with the Coconut Oil Detox (page 195).

Sjogren's Syndrome

Sjogren's syndrome is an autoimmune disease that is characterized by chronically dry eyes and mouth. Dry eyes can be eased considerably by apply 1-2 drops of coconut oil directly into the eyes. *See also* Eye Disorders. Dry mouth can be helped by drinking coconut water, which effectively hydrates the body.

Sore Throat

Take two tablespoons of the Sore Throat Syrup (page 203) every hour or two. Drink plenty of water and take 1000 mg of vitamin C and 3 to 4 tablespoons of coconut oil daily. Massage coconut oil into neck and chest.

Sprains

To reduce swelling and pain apply ice to the injured area as soon as possible. Keep the ice on for 15 minutes, then allow a 15 minute break. Repeat several times. Gently massage warm coconut oil deep into injured area. Reapply 4 to 8 times a day or use a coconut oil bandage as described on page 164. You can also use the Bone, Joint, and Cartilage Ointment on page 205.

Stretch Marks

For pregnant women, the best way to eliminate stretch marks is before the birth of the baby. Apply coconut oil to the abdomen, hips, and groin daily before delivery, but can still be effective even if started soon after delivery. Continue after delivery until abdomen is back to normal. Coconut oil or other coconut products should be eaten in the diet daily.

Stroke

See Heart Disease.

Sunburn

Gently massage coconut oil into sunburned skin. Reapply as often as necessary. To avoid sunburn, apply the oil before getting sun exposure. It is a good idea to build up tolerance to the sun by getting a little sun exposure with coconut oil every day. Gradually increase the amount of time you spend in the sun each day. Add coconut oil into the diet at the same time. Consuming the oil on a regular basis will also increase your tolerance to the sun.

Tendonitis

Activities that involve repetitive movements such as racquet sports, running, or gardening can cause tendonitis or inflammation of the tendon. Take 100 mg of grape seed extract twice a day for up to three weeks and then drop down to a maintenance dose of 50 mg. Between meals take 250 mg of bromelain (an enzyme derived from pineapple) three times daily. The Arthritis Ginger Tea (page 202) may also help relieve inflammation. Massage warm coconut oil into affected area.

Thrush

Thrush is an oral overgrowth of candida. It often occurs in infants. To treat infant thrush give the baby coconut oil. You can do this by applying the oil to the nipple when nursing or dip your finger in the oil and allow the baby to suck on it. For children over the age of 5 and adults using coconut oil to brush the teeth and for oil pulling is quite effective, *see* Gum Disease and Tooth Decay.

Toenail and Foot Fungus

Toenail fungus can be identified by yellow or brown, thick, disfigured toenails. Foot fungus is evidenced by excessively dry skin, thick calluses, and deep cracks or grooves in the skin of the foot. Foot odor is generally strong. Inflammation may also be present. Wash the feet thoroughly and dry. Massage coconut oil into the infected area and work it deep into the skin or toenail. Cover infected area in bandage soaked in coconut oil as described on page 164. If you can't keep the bandage on during the entire day at least have it on at home in the evening and while you are sleeping. Wash the feet every day with soap and water and apply a new bandage. Sunlight can be of great help too. Sunlight kills fungus. Expose the infected areas of the feet to direct sunlight for at least 20 minutes every day for about two weeks. The best time to do this is between 10:00 am and 4:00 pm when the sun is directly overhead. You should see a noticeable improvement within a week. This is most effective during the summer when the sun's rays are most intense. If you live at a latitude below 40 degrees, you should have enough sun to do this to be effective for all but the three months of winter. The coconut oil bandage may be able to get rid of the fungus by itself. Nail fungus is notoriously difficult to cure, even with drugs and medicated creams. So if possible, combine both the coconut oil and the sunbathing for best results. Depending on where you live, if it is wintertime, you may have to wait until spring to take advantage of the sun or you may go to a tanning salon. For a stronger effect, you may also use Oregano Ointment (page 204) in place of the coconut oil.

If foot or toenail fungus remains after treatment or re-occurs, it may due to a systemic candida infection. Until you solve the systemic infection, you will never be free from problems. The Coconut Oil Detox (page 195) is the best approach to this problem.

Tooth Decay

See Gum Disease and Tooth Decay.

Ulcer

Gastric ulcers are caused by bacteria burrowing into the lining of the stomach. The MCFAs in coconut can kill these organisms. Take the maintenance or therapeutic dose of coconut oil as described on pages 168 to 169. Add cayenne pepper, as much as you can tolerate, to your foods. If you don't like hot foods, you can buy cayenne in gelatin capsules and take one or two with each meal. You can get gelatin capsules at pharmacies or health food stores.

If the ulcer continues after doing the above, you should consider going on the Coconut Oil Detox (page 195).

Ulcerative Colitis

See Colon Health.

Urinary Tract Infection

Drink 6 to 8 glasses of water and consume at least 3½ tablespoons of coconut oil daily. Divide the oil throughout the day. Start doing this the moment you suspect an infection coming on. The earlier you start treatment, the quicker the problem will be resolved. At the same time, you may also drink cranberry juice. The active ingredients in cranberry juice that protects against urinary tract infections are a group of powerful antioxidants called proanthocyanidins. These antioxidants are also found in grape seeds. Proanthocyanidins can be purchased at the health food store as dietary supplements. Look for grape seed extract, Pycnogenol, or PCO.

Varicose Veins

Massage warm coconut oil into affected area 3 to 6 times a day. Take 1000 mg of vitamin C, 100 mg of grape seed extract, and 500 mg of magnesium daily, plus 1 to 3 capsules of cayenne pepper with each meal. Drink 16 ounces of coconut water and eat 3½ tablespoons of coconut oil daily. Add more fiber to your diet, especially fresh or dried coconut meat.

Viral Illness

See Bacterial and Viral Illnesses.

Warts

Some warts can be removed by simply rubbing coconut oil into them every day. This method doesn't work for all warts. Many tend to be hard and impenetrable, keeping the oil from reaching the heart of the problem. Rough up the surface of the wart with an emery board or peel or cut off some of the dry, hard skin to open it up. Apply hydrogen peroxide. Let it dry. Massage warm coconut oil deep into skin for maximum penetration. Apply the oil 4 to 8 times daily or use an oil soaked bandage as described on page 164. Continue until the skin heals and the wart is gone.

Weight Management

Weight management is a complex problem and requires much more detail than can be given here. In brief, eat 2 to 3 tablespoons of coconut oil daily with foods. Drink 2-3 quarts of water daily. Most of the water should be consumed between meals and will help to stem appetite. Eat a healthy diet rich in fresh fruits and vegetables. Eat more high fiber foods (such as coconut) and eliminate most sweets and refined carbohydrates (white bread and rice). Start an exercise program. The most successful weight loss approach is a low-carb, high-fat diet, with coconut oil as your primary source of fat. For a complete discussion on using coconut to aid in weight loss see my book *The Coconut Ketogenic Diet*.

Wrinkles

Massage coconut oil into the skin once or twice a day. Consume coconut products and the equivalent of a maintenance dose of coconut oil daily. Avoid refined vegetable oils and tobacco and eat 9 servings of vegetables a day, but don't overeat.

Yeast Infection

A vaginal yeast infection should be treated both locally and systemically. Vaginal yeast infections are always accompanied by systemic or whole body infections. To treat the vaginal infection you will use a combination of boric acid, coconut oil, and acidophilus. Fill gelatin capsules with boric acid (available at pharmacies). Insert one capsule vaginally in the morning. In the evening, douche with warm coconut oil. Before retiring for the night insert a capsule of acidophilus. Repeat this procedure for three to seven days if treating a mild infection, and for up to two weeks for a more severe infection. The boric acid suppositories can be continued for up to a month in the case of a very severe infection, but this method is usually effective within three to seven days. Coconut oil helps soothe and heal inflamed tissues and kills candida. Boric acid helps to balance pH. Acidophilus replenishes healthy flora. To address the systemic problem see Candida Infection.

Zoonosis

Zoonosis is any infectious or parasitic disease transmitted from animals to humans. *See* Bacterial and Viral Illnesses and Intestinal Parasites.

ADDITIONAL INFORMATION
www.coconutresearchcenter.org
The Coconut Research Center is a nonprofit organization dedicated to educating the medical community and general public about the health aspects of coconut. This website contains numerous articles, current research, nutritional information, and educational resources By far the best and most accurate coconut information resource available on the Internet.

www.piccadillybooks.com
This website lists the best books currently available on coconut, diet, and related health issues. Includes English and foreign language books.

REFERENCES

Chapter 3: The Coconut Medicine Chest I

1. Kiyasu, G. Y., et al. The portal transport of absorbed fatty acids. *Journal of Biological Chemistry* 1952;199:415.
2. Greenberger, N. J. and Skillman, T. G. Medium-chain triglycerides: physiologic considerations and clinical implications. *N Engl J Med* 1969;280:1045.
3. Geliebter, A. Overfeeding with medium-chain triglycerides diet results in diminished deposition of fat. *Am J of Clin Nutr* 1983;37:104.
4. Baba, N. Enhanced thermogenesis and diminished deposition of fat in response to overfeeding with a diet containing medium chain triglycerides. *Am J of Clin Nutr* 1982;35:678.
5. Tantibhedhyangkul, P. and Hashim, S. A. Medium-chain triglyceride feeding in premature infants: effects on calcium and magnesium absorption. *Pediatrics* 1978;61(4):537.
6. Jiang, Z. M., et al. A comparison of medium-chain and long-chain triglycerides in surgical patients. *Ann Surg* 1993:217(2):175.
7. Salmon, W. D. and J. G. Goodman. *J. Nutr.* 1937;13:477. Quoted by Kaunitz, H. Nutritional properties of coconut oil. *APCC Quarterly Supplement* 30 December 1971, p 35-57.
8. Cunningham, H. M. and J. K. Lossli. *Dairy Sci* 1953; 453. Quoted by Kaunitz, H. Nutritional properties of coconut oil. *APCC Quarterly Supplement* 30 December 1971, p 35-57.
9. Dutta, N. C. *Ann Biochem Expt Med* 1948; 8:69. Quoted by Kaunitz, H. Nutritional properties of coconut oil. *APCC Quarterly Supplement* 30 December 1971, p 35-57.
10. Sadasivan, V. *Current Sci* 1950;19:28. Quoted by Kaunitz, H. Nutritional properties of coconut oil. *APCC Quarterly Supplement* 30 December 1971, p 35-57.
11. Vaidya, U. V., et al. Vegetable oil fortified feeds in the nutrition of very low birthweight babies. *Indian Pediatr* 1992;29(12):1519.
12. Francois, C. A., et al. Acute effects of dietary fatty acids on the fatty acids of human milk. *Am J Clin Nutr* 1998;67:301.

13. Intengan, C. L. I. et al. Structured lipid of coconut and corn oils vs. soybean oil in the rehabilitation of malnourished children: a field study. *Philipp J Intern Med* 1992;30(30):159-164.

14. Fushiki, T. and Matsumoto, K. Swimming endurance capacity of mice is increased by chronic consumption of medium-chain triglycerides. *Journal of Nutrition* 1995;125:531.

15. Applegate, L. Nutrition. *Runner's World* 1996;31:26.

16. Stubbs, R. J. and Harbron, C.G. Covert manipulation of the ration of medium- to long-chain triglycerides in isoenergetically dense diets: effect on food intake in ad libitum feeding men. *Int. J. Obs* 1996;20:435-444.

17. Scalfi, L., et al. Postprandial thermogenesis in lean and obese subjects after meals supplemented with medium-chain and long-chain triglycerides. *Am J Clin Nutr* 1991;53:1130-1133.

18. Dulloo, A. G., et al. Twenty-four-hour energy expenditure and urinary catecholamines of humans consuming low-to-moderate amounts of medium-chain triglycerides: a dose-response study in a human respiratory chamber. *Eur J Clin Nutr* 1996;50(3):152-158.

19. St-Onge, M. and Jones, P. J. H. Physiological effects of medium-chain triglycerides: potential agents in the prevention of obesity. *J of Nutr* 2002;132(3):329-332.

20. Sadeghi, S., et al. Dietary lipids modify the cytokine response to bacterial lipopolysaccharide in mice. *Immunology* 1999;96(3):404-410.

21. Isaacs, C. E. and Thormar, H. The role of milk-derived antimicrobial lipids as antiviral and antibacterial agents in Immunology of Milk and the Neonate (Mestecky, J., et al., Eds) 1991 Plenum Press.

22. Bergsson, G., et al. Killing of Gram-positive cocci by fatty acids and monoglycerides. *APMIS* 2001;109(10):670-678.

23. Wan, J. M. and Grimble, R. F. Effect of dietary linoleate content on the metabolic response of rats to Escherichia coli endotoxin. *Clinical Science* 1987;72(3):383-385.

24. Bergsson, G., et al. In vitro inactivation of Chlamydia trachomatis by fatty acids and monoglycerides. *Antimicrobial Agents and Chemotherapy* 1998;42:2290.

25. Holland, K. T., et al. The effect of glycerol monolaurate on growth of, and production of toxic shock syndrome toxin-1 and lipase by Staphylococcus aureus. *Journal of Antimicrobial Chemotherapy* 1994;33:41.

26. Petschow, B. W., Batema, B. P., and Ford, L. L. Susceptibility of Helicobacter pylori to bactericidal properties of medium-chain monoglycerides and free fatty acids. *Antimicrob Agents Chemother* 1996;40:302-306.

27. Wang, L. L. and Johnson, E. A. Inhibition of Listeria monocytogenes by fatty acids and monoglycerides. *Appli Environ Microbiol* 1992; 58:624-629.

28. Bergsson, G., et al. In vitro killing of Candida albicans by fatty acids and monoglycerides. *Antimicrob Agents Chemother* 2001;45(11):3209-3212.

29. Isaacs, E. E., et al. Inactivation of enveloped viruses in human bodily fluids by purified lipid. *Annals of the New York Academy of Sciences* 1994;724:457.

30. Hierholzer, J. C. and Kabara, J.J. In vitro effects of monolaurin compounds on enveloped RNA and DNA viruses. *Journal of Food Safety* 1982;4:1.

31. Thormar, H., et al. Inactivation enveloped viruses and killing of cells by fatty acids and monoglycerides. *Antimicrobial Agents and Chemotherapy* 1987;31:27.

32. Kabara, J. J. *The Pharmacological Effect of Lipids.* Champaign, Ill: The American Oil Chemists' Society, 1978.

33. Issacs C. E., et al. Antiviral and antibacterial lipids in human milk and infant formula feeds. *Archives of Disease in Childhood* 1990;65:861-864.

34. Issacs, C. E., et al. Membrane-disruptive effect of human milk: inactivation of enveloped viruses. *Journal of Infectious Diseases* 1986;154:966-971.

35. Issacs, C. E., et al. Inactivation of enveloped viruses in human bodily fluids by purified lipids. *Annals of the New York Academy of Sciences* 1994;724:457-464.

36. Reiner, D. S., et al. Human milk kills Giardia lamblia by generating toxic lipolytic products. *Journal of Infectious Diseases* 1986;154:825.

37. Crouch, A. A., et al. Effect of human milk and infant milk formulae on adherence of Giardia intestinalis. *Transactions of the Royal Society of Tropical Medicine and Hygiene* 1991;85:617.

38. Chowhan, G. S., et al. Treatment of Tapeworm infestation by coconut (Concus nucifera) preparations. *Association of Physicians of India Journal.* 1985;33:207.

39. Sutter, F., et al. Comparative evaluation of rumen-protected fat, coconut oil and various oilseeds supplemented to fattening bulls. 1. Effects on growth, carcass and meat quality. *Arch. Tierernahr.* 2000;53(1):1-23.

40. Chowhan, G. S., et al. Treatment of tapeworm infestation by coconut (Cocos-nucifera) preparations. *J. Assoc. Physicians India* 1985;33(3):207-209.

41. Dayrit, C. S. Coconut Oil in Health and Disease: Its and Monolaurin's Potential as Cure for HIV/AIDS. Paper presented at the 37th Annual Cocotech Meeting, Chennai, India, July 25, 2000.

42. Witcher, K. J., et al. Modulation of immune cell proliferation by glycerol monolaurate. *Clin Diagn Lab Immunol* 1996;3(1):10-13.

43. Pimentel, M., et al. Normalization of lactulose breath testing correlates with symptom improvement in irritable bowel syndrome: a double-blind, randomized, placebo-controlled study. *Am J Gastroenterol* 2003;98(2):412-419.

44. Kono, H., et al. Medium-chain triglycerides enhance secretory IgA expression in rat intestine after administration of endotoxin. *Am J Physiol Gastrointest Liver Physiol* 2004;286:G1081-1089.

45. Arranza, J. L. The Dietary Fat Produced in Asian Countries and Human Health. Paper presented at the 7th Asian Congress of Nutrition in Beijing, October 8, 1995.

46. Vitamin E and melanoma. *Free Radical Biology and Medicine* 1997;7(22). Cited in *Life Extension* Nov. 1997, p 30.

47. Passwater, R. A. *The Antioxidants*. New Canaan, CT: Keats Publishing, 1985, p 10-11.

48. Burk, K., et al. The effects of topical and oral I-selenomethionine on pigmentation and skin cancer incidence by ultraviolet irradiation. *Nutrition and Cancer* 1992;17:123.

49. Delver, E. and Pence, B. Effects of dietary selenium level on uv-induced skin cancer and epidermal antioxidant status. *FASEB Journal* 1993;7:A290.

50. Epstein, J. H. Effects of beta-carotene on ultraviolet induced cancer formation in the Harless mouse skin. *Photochem Photobiol* 1977;25:211.

51. *Life Extension*. December 1997, p 5-8.

52. Hopkins, G. J., et al. Polyunsaturated fatty acids as promoters of mammary carcinogenesis induced in Sprague-Dawley rats by 7, 12-dimethylbenz[a] anthracene. *J Natl Cancer Inst.* 1981;66(3):517.

53. Seddon, J. M., et al. Progression of age-related macular degeneration: association with dietary fat, transunsaturated fat, nuts, and fish intake. *Arch Ophthalmol* 2003;121(12):1728-1737.

54. Ouchi, M., et al. A novel relation of fatty acid with age-related macular degeneration. *Ophthalmologica* 2002;216(5):363-367.

55. Seddon, J. M., et al. Dietary fat and risk for advanced age-related macular degeneration. *Arch Ophthalmol* 2001;119(8):1191-1199.

56. Ross, D. L., et al. Early biochemical and EEG correlates of the ketogenic diet in children with atypical absence epilepsy. *Pediatr Neurol* 1985;1(2):104.

57. Brod, J., et al. Evolution of lipid composition in skin treated with black currant seed oil. *Int J Cosmetic Sci* 1988;10:149.

58. Reddy, B. S. and Maeura, Y. Tumor promotion by dietary fat in azoxymethane-induced colon carcinogenesis in female F344 rats: influence of amount and source of dietary fat. *J Natl Cancer Inst* 1984;72(3):745-750.

59. Cohen, L. A. and Thompson, D.O. The influence of dietary medium chain triglycerides on rat mammary tumor development. *Lipids* 1987;22(6):455-461.

60. Cohen, L. A., et al. Influence of dietary medium-chain triglycerides on the development of N-methylnitrosourea-induced rat mammary tumor. *Cancer Res* 1984;44(11):5023-5028.

61. Nolasco, N. A., et al. Effect of Coconut oil, trilaurin and tripalmitin on the promotion stage of carcinogenesis. *Philipp J Sci* 1994;123(1):161-169.

62. Bulatao-Jayme, J., et al. Epdemiology of primary liver cancer in the Philippines with special consideration of a possible aflatoxin factor. *J Philipp Med Assoc* 1976;52(5-6):129-150.

63. Ling, P. R., et al. Structured lipid made from fish oil and medium-chain triglycerides alters tumor and host metabolism in Yoshida-sarcoma-bearing rats. *Am J Clin Nutr* 1991;53(5):1177-1184.

64. Holleb, A. I. *The American Cancer Society Cancer Book*. New York: Doubleday & Company, 1986.

65. Witcher, K. J., et al. Modulation of immune cell proliferation by glycerol monolaurate. *Clinical and Diagnostic Laboratory Immunology* 1996;3:10-13.

66. Ling, P. R., et al. Structured lipid made from fish oil and medium-chain triglycerides alters tumor and host metabolism in Yoshida-sarcoma-bearing rats. *Am J Clin Nutr* 1991;53(5):1177-1184.

67. Kono, H., et al. Medium-chain triglycerides inhibit free radical formation and TNF-alpha production in rats given enteral ethanol. *Am J Physiol Gastrointest Liver Physiol* 2000;278(3):G467.

68. Cha, Y. S. and Sachan, D.S. Opposite effects of dietary saturated and unsaturated fatty acids on ethanol-pharmacokinetics, triglycerides and carnitines. *J Am Coll Nutr* 1994;13(4):338.

69. Nanji, A. A., et al. Dietary saturated fatty acids: a novel treatment for alcoholic liver disease. *Gastroenterology* 1995;109(2):547.

70. Trocki, O. Carnitine supplementation vs. medium-chain triglycerides in postburn nutritional support. *Burns Incl Therm Inj* 1988;14(5):379-387.

71. Moore, S. Thrombosis and atherogenesis—the chicken and the egg: contribution of platelets in atherogenesis. *Ann NY Acad Sci* 1985;454:146-153.

72. Stewart, J. W., et al. Effect of various triglycerides on blood and tissue cholesterol of calves. *J Nutr* 1978;108:561-566.

73. Awad, A. B. Effect of dietary lipids on composition and glucose utilization by rat adipose tissue. *Journal of Nutrition* 1981;111:34-39.

74. Monserrat, A. J., et al. Protective effect of coconut oil on renal necrosis occurring in rats fed a methyl-deficient diet. *Ren Fail* 1995;17(5):525.

75. Skrzydlewska, E., et al. Antioxidant status and lipid peroxidation in colorectal cancer. *J Toxicol Environ Health A* 2001;64(3):213-222.

76. Witcher, K. J., et al. Modulation of immune cell proliferation by glycerol monolaurate. *Clinical and Diagnostic Laboratory Immunology* 1996;3:10-13.

77. Bulatao-Jayme, J., et al. Epdemiology of primary liver cancer in the Philippines with special consideration of a possible aflatoxin factor. *J Philipp Med Assoc* 1976;52(5-6):129-150.

78. Nolasco, N. A., et al. Effect of Coconut oil, trilaurin and tripalmitin on the promotion stage of carcinogenesis. *Philipp J Sci* 1994;123(1):161-169.

79. Kono, H. et al. Medium-chain triglycerides enhance secretory IgA expression in rat intestine after administration of endotoxin. *Am J Physiol Gastrointest Liver Physiol* 2004;286:G1081-1089.

80. Dave, J. R., et al. Dodecylglycerol provides partial protection against glutamate toxicity in neuronal cultures derived from different regions of embryonic rat brain. *Mol Chem Neuropathol* 1997;30:1-13.

81. Blaylock, R. L., MD, *Excitoxins: The Taste that Kills*. Santa Fe, NM: Health Press 1994, p19.

82. Reddy, B. S. and Maeura, Y. Tumor promotion by dietary fat in azoxymethane-induced colon carcinogenesis in female F344 rats: influence of amount and source of dietary fat. *J Natl Cancer Inst* 1984;72(3):745-750.

83. Cohen, L. A. and Thompson, D. O. The influence of dietary medium chain triglycerides on rat mammary tumor development. *Lipids* 1987;22(6):455-461.

84. Lim-Sylianco, C. Y., et al. A comparison of germ cell antigenotoxic activity of non-dietary and dietary coconut oil and soybean oil. *Phil J of Coconut Studies* 1992;2:1-5.

85. Lim-Sylianco, C. Y., et al. Antigenotoxic effects of bone marrow cells of coconut oil versus soybean oil. *Phil J of Coconut Studies.* 1992;2:6-10.

86. Witcher, K. J, et al. Modulation of immune cell proliferation by glycerol monolaurate. *Clinical and Diagnostic Laboratory Immunology* 1996;3:10-13.

87. Projan, S. J., et al. Glyceryl monolaurate inhibits the production of β-lactamase, toxic shock syndrome toxin-1 and other Staphylococcal exoproteins by interfering with signal transduction. *J of Bacteriol.* 1994;176:4204:4209.

88. Teo, T. C., et al. Long-term feeding with structured lipid composed of medium-chain and N-3 fatty acids ameliorates endotoxic shock in guinea pigs. *Metabolism* 1991;40(1):1152-1159.

89. Lim-Navarro, P. R. T. Protection effect of coconut oil against E coli endotoxin shock in rats. *Coconuts Today* 1994;11:90-91.

90. Garland, F. C., et al. Occupational sunlight exposure and melanoma in the U.S. Navy. *Archives of Environmental Health* 1990;*45*:261-267.

91. Feldman, D., et al, Vitamin D and prostate cancer. *Endocrinology* 2000;141:5-9.

92. Billaudel B., et al. Vitamin D3 deficiency and alterations of glucose metabolism in rat endocrine pancreas. *Diabetes Metab* 1998;24:344-350.

93. Bourlon, P. M., et al. Influence of vitamin D3 deficiency and 1, 225 dihydroxyvitamin D3 on de novo insulin biosynthesis in the islets of the rat endocrine pancreas. *J Endocrinol* 1999;160:87-95.

94. Ortlepp, J. R., et al. The vitamin D receptor gene variant is associated with the prevalence of type 2 diabetes mellitus and coronary artery disease. *Diabet Med* 18(10):842-845.

95. Hypponen E., et al. Intake of vitamin D and risk of type 1 diabetes: a birth-cohort study. *Lancet* 2001;358(9292):1500-1503.

96. Bouillon R., et al. Polyunsaturated fatty acids decrease the apparent affinity of vitamin D metabolites for human vitamin D-binding protein. *J Steroid Biochem Mol Biol* 1992;42:855-861.

97. Reger, M.A., et al. Effects of beta-hydroxybutyrate on cognition in memory-impaired adults. *Neurobiol Aging* 2004;25:311-314.

98. Nafar, F. and Mearow, K.M. Coconut oil attenuates the effects of amyloid-beta on cortical neurons in vitro. *J Alzheimers Dis* 2014;39:233-237.

Chapter 4: Coconut Oil On Trial

1. Hashim, S. A., et al. Effect of mixed fat formula feeding on serum cholesterol level in man. *Am J of Clin Nutr* 1959;7:30-34.

2. Bierenbaum, J. L., et al. Modified-fat dietary management of the young male with coronary disease: a five-year report. *JAMA* 1967;202:1119-1123.

3. Prior, I. A., et al. Cholesterol, coconuts and diet in Polynesian atolls—a natural experiment; the Pukapuka and Toklau island studies. *Am J Clin Nutr* 1981;34:1552-1561.

4. Hegsted, D. M., et al. Qualitative effects of dietary fat on serum cholesterol in man. *Am J of Clin Nutr* 1965;17:281.

5. Kintanar, Q. L. Is coconut oil hypercholesterolemic and atherogenic? A focused review of the literature. *Trans Nat Acad Science and Techn (Phil)* 1988;10:371-414.

6. Blackburn, G. L., et al. A reevaluation of coconut oil's effect on serum cholesterol and atherogenesis. *J Philipp Med Assoc* 1989;65(1):144-152.

7. Kaunitz, H. and Dayrit, C. S. Coconut oil consumption and coronary heart disease. *Philipp J Intern Med* 1992;30:165-171.

8. Wojcicki, J., et al. A search for a model of experimental atherosclerosis: comparative studies in rabbits, guinea pigs and rats. *Pol J Pharmacol Pharm* 1985;37(1):11-21.

9. Lin, M. H., et al. Lipoprotein responses to fish, coconut and soybean oil diets with and without cholesterol in the Syrian hamster. *J Formos Med Assoc* 1995;94(12):724-731.

10. Ahrens, E. H. Nutritional factors and serum lipid levels. *Am J Med* 1957;23:928.

11. Hu, F. B., et al. Dietary fat intake and the risk of coronary heart disease in women, *N. Engl J Med* 1997; 337:1491-1499.

12. Willett, W. C., et al. Intake of trans-fatty acids and risk of coronary heart disease among women. *Lancet* 1993;341:581-585.

13. Ascherio, A., et al. Trans fatty acids and coronary heart disease. *N. Engl J Med* 1999; 340:1994-1998.

14. de Roos, N. M., et al. Consumption of a solid fat rich in lauric acid results in a more favorable serum lipid profile in healthy men and women than consumption of a solid fat rich in trans-fatty acids. *J Nutr* 2001;131:242-245.

15. Williams, M. A., et al. Increased plasma triglyceride secretion in EFA-deficient rats fed diets with or without saturated fat. *Lipids* 1989;24(5):448-453.

16. Morin, R. J., et al. Effects of essential fatty acid deficiency and supplementation on atheroma formation and regression. *J Atheroscler Res* 1964;4:387-396.

15. McCullagh, K. G., et al. Experimental canine atherosclerosis and its prevention. *Lab Invest* 1976;34:394-405.

16. Yamamoto, Y. and Muramatsu, K. Regulation of essential fatty acid intake in the rat: self-selection of corn oil. *J Nutr Sci Vitaminol (Tokyo)* 1988;34(1):107-116.

17. Cater, N. B., et al. Comparison of the effects of medium-chain triacylglycerols, palm oil, and high oleic acid sunflower oil on plasma triacylglycerol fatty acids and lipid and lipoprotein concentrations in humans. *Am J Clin Nutr* 1997;65(1):41-45.

18. Calabrese, C., et al. A cross-over study of the effect of a single oral feeding of medium chain triglyceride oil vs. canola oil on post-ingestion plasma triglyceride levels in healthy me. *Altern Med Rev* 1999;4(1):23-28.

19. Bourque, C., et al. Consumption of oil composed of medium chain triacyglycerols, phytosterols, and N-3 fatty acids improves cardiovascular risk profile in overweight women. *Metabolism* 2003;52(6):771-777.

20. Ng, T. K. W., et al. Nonhypercholesterolemic effects of a palm-oil diet in Malaysian volunteers. *Am J Clin Nutr* 1991;53:1552-1561.

21. Tholstrup, T., et al. Fat high in stearic acid favorably affects blood lipids and factor VII coagulant activity in comparison with fats high in palmitic acid or high in myristic and lauric acids. *Am J Clin Nutr* 1994;59:371-377.

22. Keys, A. Coronary heart disease in seven countries. *Circulation* 1970;41;Suppl 1:1-211.

23. Kaunitz, H. and Dayrit, C. S. Coconut oil consumption and coronary heart disease. *Phili J Inter Med* 1992;30:165-171.

24. Dayrit, C. S. Coconut Oil: atherogenic or not? *Philippine Journal of Cardiology* 2003;31:97-104.

Chapter 5: Coconut Oil Is Good for Your Heart

1. Shorland, F. B., et al. Studies on fatty acid composition of adipose tissue and blood lipids of Polynesians. *Am J Clin Nutr* 1969;22(5):594-605.

2. Prior, I. A. M., et al. Cholesterol, coconuts, and diet on Polynesian atolls: a natural experiment: the Pukapuka and Tokelau Island studies. *Am J Clin Nutr* 1981;34:1552.

3. Misch, K. A. Ischaemic heart disease in urbanized Papua New Guinea. An autopsy study. *Cardiology* 1988;75(1):71-75.

4. Lindeberg, S. Age relations of cardiovascular risk factors in a traditional Melanesian society; the Kitava Study. *Am J Clin Nutr* 1997;66(4):845-852.

5. Lindeberg, S. and Lundh, B. Apparent absence of stroke and ischaemic heart disease in a traditional Melanesian island: a clinical study in Kitava. *J Intern Med* 1993;233(3):269-275.

6. Lindeberg, S., et al. Cardiovascular risk factors in a Melanesian population apparently free from stroke and ischaemic heart disease; the Kitava study. *J Intern Med* 1994;236(3):331-340.

7. Mendis, S. Coronary heart disease and coronary risk profile in a primitive population. *Trop Geogr Med* 1991;43(1-2):199-202.

8. Dayrit, C. S. Coconut oil: atherogenic or not? *Philip J Cardiology* 2003;31(3):97-104.

9. Lindeberg, S., et al. Low serum insulin in traditional Pacific Islanders—the Kitava Study. *Metabolism* 1999;48(10):1216-1219.

10. Prior, I. A. M. The price of civilization. *Nutrition Today*, July/Aug 1971, p 2-11.

11. Stanhope, J. M., et al. The Tokelau Island migrant study: serum lipid concentrations in two environments. *J Chron Dis* 1981;34:45.

12. Kannel, W. B., et al. Cholesterol in the prediction of atherosclerotic disease. New perspectives based on the Framingham study. *Annals of Internal Medicine* 1979;90:85-91.

13. Hong, M. K., et al. Usefulness of the total cholesterol to high-density lipoprotein cholesterol ratio in predicting angiographic coronary artery disease in women. *Am J Cardiol* 1991;15;68(17):1646-1650.

14. Mensink, R. P., et al. Effects of dietary fatty acids and carbohydrates on the ratio of serum total to HDL cholesterol and on serum lipids and apolipoproteins: a meta-analysis of 60 controlled trials. *Am J Clin Nutr* 2003; 77(5):1146-1155.

15. Temme, E. H. M., et al. Comparison of the effects of diets enriched in lauric, palmitic or oleic acids on serum lipids and lipoproteins in healthy men and women. *Am J Clin Nutr* 1996;63:897-903.

16. Zock, P. L., and Katan, M. B. Hydrogenation alternatives: Effects of trans-fatty acids and stearic acid versus linoleic acid on serum lipids and lipoproteins in humans. *J Lipid Res* 1992;33:399-410.

17. de Roos, N. M., et al. Consumption of a solid fat rich in lauric acid results in a more favorable serum lipid profile in healthy men and women than consumption of a solid fat rich in trans-fatty acids. *J Nutr* 2001;131:242-245.

18. Sundram, K., et al. Trans (elaidic) fatty acids adversely affect the lipoprotein profile relative to specific saturated fatty acids in humans. *J Nutr* 1997;127:514S-520S.

19. Mensink, R. P., and Katan, M. B. Effect of dietary fatty acids on serum lipids and lipoproteins. A meta- analysis of 27 trials. *Arteriosclerosis, Thrombosis, and Vascular Biology* 1992;12;911-919.

20. Mendis, S., et al. The effects of replacing coconut oil with corn oil on human serum lipid profiles and platelet derived factors active in atherogenesis. *Nutrition Reports International* Oct. 1989;40(4).

21. Hostmark, A. T., et al. Plasma lipid concentration and liver output of lipoproteins in rats fed coconut fat or sunflower oil. *Artery* 1980;7:367-383.

22. Arranza, J. L. *The Dietary Fat Produced in Asian Countries and Human Health*. Paper presented at the 7th Asian Congress of Nutrition in Beijing, October 08, 1995.

23. Bach, A. C. and Babayan, V. K. Medium chain triglycerides: an update. *Am J Clin Nutr* 1982;36:960-962.

24. Garfinkel, M., et al. 1992. Insulinotropic potency of lauric acid: a metabolic rationale for medium chain fatty acids (MCF) in TPN formulation. *J Surg Res* 52:328-333.

25. Han, J., et al. Medium-chain oil reduces fat mass and down-regulates expression of adipogenic genes in rats. *Obes Res* 2003;11(6):734-744.

26. Trinidad, T. P., et al. Glycaemic index of different coconut (Cocos nucifera)-flour products in normal and diabetic subjects. *British Journal of Nutrition* 2003;90:551-556.

27. Prior, I. A. M., et al. Cholesterol, coconuts, and diet on Polynesian atolls: a natural experiment: the Pukapuka and Tokelau Island studies. *Am J Clin Nutr* 1981;34:1552.

28. Lindeberg, S., et al. Low serum insulin in traditional pacific Islanders—the Kitava Study. *Metabolism* 1999;48(10):1216-1219.

29. Larsen, L. F., et al. Effects of dietary fat quality and quantity on postprandial activation of blood coagulation factor VII. *Arterioscler Thromb Vasc Biol.* 1997; 17(11):2904-2909.

30. McGregor, L. Effects of feeding with hydrogenated coconut oil on platelet function in rats. *Proc Nutr Soc* 1974;33:1A-2A.

31. Vas Dias, F. W., et al. The effect of polyunsaturated fatty acids of the n-3 and n-6 series on platelet aggregation and platelet and aortic fatty acid composition in rabbits. *Atherosclerosis* 1982;43:245-57.

32. Ferrannini, E., et al. Insulin resistance in essential hypertension, *New Engl J of Med* 1987;317:350-357.

33. Hunter, T. D. *Fed Proc* 21, Suppl. 1962;11:36 Quoted by Kaunitz, H. Nutritional properties of coconut oil. *APCC Quarterly Supplement* 30 December 1971, p 35-57.

34. Lindeberg, S., et al. Low serum insulin in traditional Pacific Islanders—the Kitava Study. *Metabolism* 1999;48(10):1216-1219.

35. Verhoef, P., et al. Plasma total homocysteine, B vitamins, and risk of coronary atherosclerosis. *Arteriosclerosis, Thrombosis, and Vascular Biology* 1997;17:989-995.

36. Ridker, P., et al. C-reactive protein and other markers of inflammation in the prediction of cardiovascular disease in women. *N Engl J Med* 2000;342(12):836-843.

37. Simon, H. B. Patient-directed, nonprescription approaches to cardiovascular disease. *Arch Intern Med* 1994;154(20):2283-2296.

38. Felton, C. V., et al. Dietary polyunsaturated fatty acids and composition of human aortic plaques. *Lancet* 1994;344:1195-1196.

39. Morrison, H. I., et al. Periodontal disease and risk of fatal coronary heart and cerebrovascular diseases. *J Cardiovasc Risk* 1999;6(1):7-11.

40. Loesche, W., et al. Assessing the relationship between dental disease and coronary heart disease in elderly U.S. veterans. *J Am Dent Assoc* 1998;129(3):301-311.

41. Raza-Ahmad, A., et al. Evidence of type 2 herpes simplex infection in human coronary arteries at the time of coronary artery bypass surgery. *Can J Cardiol* 1995;11(11):1025-1029.

42. Imaizumi, M., et al. Risk for ischemic heart disease and all-cause mortality in subclinical hypothyroidism. *J Clin Endocrinol Metab* 2004;89(7):3365-3370.

Chapter 6: The Coconut Medicine Chest II

1. Burkitt, D. P. Hiatus Hernia: Is it preventable? *Am J Clin Nutr* 1981;34:428-431.

2. Jewell, D. R. and Jewell, C.T. *The Oat and Wheat Bran Health Plan.* New York: Bantam Books, 1989.

3. Rose, D. P., et al. High-fiber diet reduces serum estrogen concentrations in premenopausal women. *Am J Clin Nutr* 1991;54:520-525.

4. Manoj, G., et al. Effect of dietary fiber on the activity of intestinal and fecal beta-glucuronidase activity during 1, 2-dimethylhydrazine induced colon carcinogenesis. *Plant Foods Hum Nutr* 2001;56(1):13-21.

5. Kabara, J. J. *The Pharmacological Effect of Lipids.* Champaign, Ill: The American Oil Chemists' Society, 1978.

6. Harig, J. M., et al. Treatment of diversion colitis with short-chain-fatty acids irrigation. *N Engl J Med* 1989;320(1):23-28.

7. Eyton, A. *The F-Plan Diet.* New York: Crown Publisher, Inc. 1983.

8. Lindeberg, S., et al. Age relations of cardiovascular risk factors in a traditional Melanesian society; the Kitava Study. *Am J Clin Nutr* 1997;66(4):845-852.

9. Anderson, J. W. and Gustafson, N. J. Type II diabetes: current nutrition management concepts. *Geriatrics* 1986;41:28-35.

10. Sindurani, J. A. and Rajamohan, T. Effects of different levels of coconut fiber on blood glucose, serum insulin and minerals in rats. *Indian J Physiol Pharmacol* 2000;44(1):97-100.

11. Trinidad, T. P., et al. Glycaemic index of different coconut (Cocos nucifera)-flour products in normal and diabetic subjects. *British Journal of Nutrition* 2003;90:551-556.

12. Liu, S., et al. Whole-grain consumption and risk of coronary heart disease: results from the Nurses' Health Study. *Am J Clin Nutr* 1999;70:412-419.

13. Rimm, E. B., et al. Vegetable, fruit, and cereal fiber intake and risk of coronary heart disease among men. *JAMA* 1996;275(6):447-451.

14. Liu, S., et al. Whole grain consumption and risk of ischemic stroke in women: A prospective study. *JAMA* 2000;284(12):1534-1540.

15. Anderson, J. W. and Gustafson, N. J. *Dr. Anderson's High-Fiber Fitness Plan.* Lexington, Kentucky: The University Press of Kentucky, 1994.

16. Cummings, J. H. Dietary Fibre. *British Medical Bulletin* 1981;37:65-70.

17. Song, Y. J., et al. Soluble dietary fibre improves insulin sensitivity by increasing muscle GLUT-4 content in stroke-prone spontaneously hypertensive rats. *Clin Exp Pharmacol Physiol* 2000;27(1-2):41-45.

18. Ludwig, D. S., et al. Dietary fiber, weight gain, and cardiovascular disease risk factors in young adults. *JAMA* 1999;282:1539-1546.

19. Salil, G. and Rajamohan, T. Hypolipidemic and antiperoxidative effect of coconut protein in hypercholesterolemic rats. *Indian J Exp Biol* 2001;39(10):1028-1034.

20. Padmakumaran Nair, K. G., et al. Coconut kernel protein modifies the effect of coconut oil on serum lipids. *Plant Foods Hum. Nutr* 1999;53(2):133-144.

21. Salil, G. and Rajamohan, T. Hypolipidemic and antiperoxidative effect of coconut protein in hypercholesterolemic rats. *Indian J Exp Biol* 2001;39(10):1028-1034.

22. Chopra, R. N. Anthelminthics acting on Cestodes. In: Mukerjee N. Ed. *A handbook of tropical therapeutics.* Calcutta Art Press. 1936, p 283.

23. Nadkarni, K. M. Cocos Nucifera. In: *Indian Materia Medica with Ayurvedic, Unani – Tibbi, sidha, Allopathic, Homeopathi and Home remedies 3rd Ed.* Bombay: Popular Prakashan. 1976, p 363-364.

24. Chowhan, G. S., et al. Treatment of tapeworm infestation by coconut (cocos-nucifera) Preparations. *Journal of the Association of Physicians of India* 1985;33(3):207-209.

25. Trinidad, P. T., et al. Nutritional and health benefits of coconut flour: study 1: The effect of coconut flour on mineral availability. *Philipp J Nutr* 2002;49(102):48-57.

26. Lupton, J. R. and Turner, N. D. Potential protective mechanisms of wheat bran fiber. *Am J Med* 1999;106(1A):24S-27S.

27. Jacobs, D. R., Jr., et al. Is whole grain intake associated with reduced total and cause-specific death rates in older women? The Iowa Women's Health Study. *Am J Public Health.* 1999;89(3):322-329.

28. Mozaffarian, D., et al. Cereal, fruit, and vegetable fiber intake and risk of cardiovascular disease in elderly individuals. *JAMA* 2003;289:1659-1666.

29. Spiller, G., and Freeman, H. Recent advances in dietary fiber and colorectal diseases. *Am J Clin Nutr* 1981;34:1145-1152.

30. Campbell-Falck, D., et al. The intravenous use of coconut water. *Am J Emerg Med* 2000;18(1):108:111.

31. Pummer, S., et al. Influence of coconut water on hemostasis. *Am J Emerg Med* 2001;19(4):287-289.

32. Anzaldo, F. E., et al. Coconut water as intravenous fluid. *Philipp J Pediatr* 1975;24(4):143-166.

33. Recio, P. M., et al. The intravenous use of coconut water. *Philipp J Surg Spec* 1974;30(30):119-140.

34. Ludan, A. C. Modified coconut water for oral rehydration. *Philipp J Pediatr* 1980;29(5):344-351.

35. Zhao, G., et al. Effects of coconut juice on the formation of hyperlipidemia and Atherosclerosis. *Chinese Journal of Preventive Medicine* 1995;29(4):216-8.

36. Macalalag, E. V., Jr. and Macalalag, A. L. Bukolysis: young coconut water renoclysis for urinary stone dissolution *Int Surg* 1987;72(4):247.

37. Poblete, G. S., et al. The effect of coconut water on intraocular pressure of normal subjects. *Philipp J Ophthal* 1999;24(1):3-5.

38. Mantena, S. K., et al. In vitro evaluation of antioxidant properties of Cocos nucifera Linn. water. *Nahrung* 2003;47(2):126-131.

39. May, C. D. Food allergy: Perspective, principles, and practical management. *Nutrition Today* Nov/Dec 1980, p 28-32.

40. Fries, J. H. and Fries, M. W. Coconut: a review of its uses as they relate to the allergic individual. *Ann Allergy* 1983;51(4):472-481.

41. Teuber, S. S. and Peterson, W. R. Systemic allergic reaction to coconut (Cocos nucifera) in 2 subjects with hypersensitivity to tree nut and demonstration of cross-reactivity to legumin-like seed storage proteins: new coconut and walnut food allergens. *J Allergy Clin Immunol* 1999;103(6):1180-1185.

42. Gan, B. S., et al. Lactobacillus fermentum RC-14 inhibits Staphylococcus aureus infection of surgical implants in rats. *J Infect Dis* 2002;185(9):1369-1372.

43. Veer, P., et al. Consumption of fermented milk products and breast cancer: a case-control study in The Netherlands. *Cancer Res* 1989;49:4020-4023.

44. Le, M. G., et al. Consumption of dairy products and alcohol in a case control study of breast cancer. *JNCI* 1986;77:633-636.

45. Biffi, A., et al. Antiproliferative effect of fermented milk on the growth of a human breast cancer cell line. *Nutrition and Cancer* 1997;28(1):93-99.

Chapter 7: How to Be Happy, Healthy, and Beautiful

1. Rele, A. S. and Mohile, R. B. Effect of mineral oil, sunflower oil, and coconut oil on prevention of hair damage. *J Cosmet Sci* 2003;54(2):175-192.

2. Kabara, J. J. *The Pharmacological Effect of Lipids.* Champaign, Ill: The American Oil Chemists' Society, 1978.

INDEX

Stop Alzheimer's Now!

How to Prevent and Reverse Dementia, Parkinson's, ALS, Multiple Sclerosis, and Other Neurodegenerative Disorders

More than 35 million people have dementia today. Each year 4.6 million new cases occur worldwide—one new case every 7 seconds. Alzheimer's disease is the most common form of dementia. Parkinson's disease, another progressive brain disorder, affects about 4 million people worldwide. Millions more suffer with other neurodegenerative disorders. The number of people affected by these destructive diseases continues to increase every year.

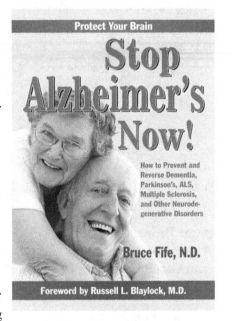

Dementia and other forms of neurodegeneration are not a part of the normal aging process. The brain is fully capable of functioning normally for a lifetime, regardless of how long a person lives. While aging is a risk factor for neurodegeneration, it is not the cause! Dementia and other neurodegenerative disorders are disease processes that can be prevented and successfully treated.

This book outlines a program using a coconut oil-based diet that is backed by decades of medical and clinical research and has proven successful in restoring mental function and improving both brain and overall health. You will learn how to prevent and even reverse symptoms associated with Alzheimer's disease, Parkinson's disease, amyotrophic lateral sclerosis (ALS), multiple sclerosis (MS), Huntington's disease, epilepsy, diabetes, stroke, and various forms of dementia.

The information in this book is useful not only for those who are suffering from neurodegenerative disease but for anyone who wants to be spared from ever encountering these devastating afflictions. These diseases don't just happen overnight. They take years, often decades, to develop. In the case of Alzheimer's disease, approximately 70 percent the brain cells responsible for memory are destroyed before symptoms become noticeable.

You can stop Alzheimer's and other neurodegenerative diseases before they take over your life. The best time to start is now.

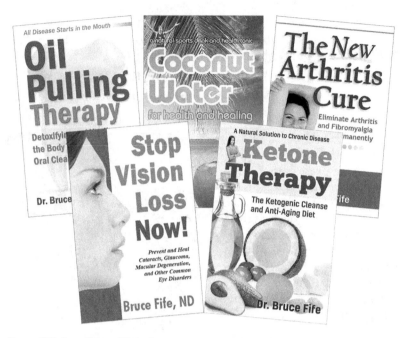

Stop Vision Loss Now!
Prevent and Heal Cataracts, Glaucoma, Macular Degeneration, and Other Common Eye Disorders

Losing your eyesight is a frightening thought, yet every five seconds, someone in the world goes blind. Most visual impairment is caused by age-related diseases, such as cataracts, glaucoma, macular degeneration, and diabetic retinopathy, all debilitating conditions for which modern medicine has no cure. However, that does not mean there is no hope. There is a successful treatment, one that does not involve surgery, drugs, or invasive medical procedures. The solution involves an innovative coconut oil-based diet.

Most chronic eye disorders strike without warning and none of us can tell who will develop a visual handicap as we age. In this book, you will learn the basic underlying causes for the most common degenerative eye disorders and what you can do to prevent, stop, and even reverse them.

The New Arthritis Cure
Eliminate Arthritis and Fibromyalgia Pain Permanently

Up until now, arthritis and fibromyalgia have been considered incurable partly because doctors do not know what causes them. Recent medical research, however, has discovered the cause in most cases. In this book you will read about new groundbreaking medical research, fascinating case studies, and inspiring personal success stories. You will lean about a totally unique approach to overcoming arthritis and fibromyalgia called the Arthritis Battle Plan. More importantly, you will earn what steps you must take in order to stop the disease process and regain your health.

Ketone Therapy
The Ketogenic Cleanse and Anti-Aging Diet

Ketones are high-potency fuel that boost energy and cellular efficiency and activates special enzymes that regulate cell survival, repair, and growth. When a person is in nutritional ketosis, blood levels of ketones are elevated to therapeutic levels. In response, high blood pressure drops, cholesterol levels improve, inflammation is reduced, blood sugar levels normalize, and overall health improves. Many health problems that are difficult to treat are quickly reversed. Medications that were once relied on daily are no longer necessary. People are discovering that a simple, but revolutionary diet based on wholesome, natural foods, and the most health-promoting fats is dramatically changing their lives.

Oil Pulling Therapy
Detoxifying and Healing the Body Through Oral Cleansing

If you have bad breath, bleeding gums, cavities, or tooth pain, you need this book! If you suffer from asthma, diabetes, arthritis, migraine headaches, or any chronic illness, and have not found relief, this book could have the solution you need.

Recent research has demonstrated a direct link between oral health and chronic illness. Simply improving the health of your teeth and gums can cure many chronic problems. Despite advances in modern dentistry, over 90 percent of the population has some level of gum disease or tooth decay. More brushing, flossing, and mouthwash isn't the solution. What will work is Oil Pulling Therapy. Oil pulling is an age-old method of oral cleansing originating from Ayurvedic medicine.

In this book, the science behind oil pulling is fully documented with references to medical studies and case histories. Although oil pulling is a very simple procedure, it is one of the most powerful and effective methods of detoxification and healing in natural medicine.

Coconut Water for Health and Healing

Coconut water is a refreshing beverage that is a powerhouse of nutrition containing a complex blend of vitamins, minerals, amino acids, antioxidants, enzymes, health-enhancing growth factors, and other phytonutrients.

Because its electrolyte (ionic mineral) content is similar to human plasma, it has gained international acclaim as a natural sports drink for oral rehydration. As such, it has proven superior to commercial sports drinks.

Coconut water's unique nutritional profile gives it the power to balance body chemistry, ward off disease, fight cancer, and retard aging. History and folklore credits coconut water with remarkable healing powers, which medical science is now confirming.

The Coconut Ketogenic Diet

Supercharge Your Metabolism, Revitalize Thyroid Function, and Lose Excess Weight

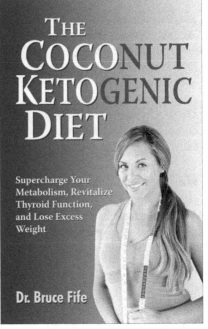

You can enjoy eating rich, full-fat foods and lose weight without counting calories or suffering from hunger. The secret is a high-fat, ketogenic diet. Our bodies need fat. It's necessary for optimal health. It's also necessary in order to lose weight safely and naturally.

Low-fat diets have been heavily promoted for the past three decades, and as a result, we are fatter now than ever before. Obviously, there is something wrong with the low-fat approach to weight loss. There is a better solution to the obesity epidemic, and that solution is The Coconut Ketogenic Diet. This book exposes many common myths and misconceptions about fats and explains why low-fat diets don't work. It also reveals new, cutting-edge research on the world's only natural low-calorie fat—coconut oil—and how you can use it to boost your energy, stimulate metabolism, improve thyroid function, and lose excess weight.

This revolutionary weight loss program is designed to keep you both slim and healthy using wholesome, natural foods, and the most health-promoting fats. It has proven successful in helping those suffering from obesity, diabetes, heart and circulatory problems, low thyroid function, chronic fatigue, high blood pressure, high cholesterol, and many other conditions.

In this book you will learn:

- Why you need to eat fat to lose fat
- Why you should not eat lean protein without a source of fat
- How to lose weight without feeling hungry or miserable
- How to stop food cravings dead cold
- Which fats promote health and which ones don't
- How to jumpstart your metabolism
- How to revitalize a sluggish thyroid
- How to use your diet to overcome common health problems
- How to reach your ideal weight and stay there
- Why eating rich, delicious foods can help you lose weight

Visit Us on the Web

P̲B̲ Piccadilly Books, Ltd.

www.piccadillybooks.com